Who I Am Yesterday

A Path to Coping With A Loved One's Dementia

Victoria Adams

Copyright © 2012 Victoria Adams

Cover design by the author

Photograph by the author: Cathedral Grove, Vancouver Island, British Columbia

All rights reserved.

ISBN: 10-1475152183
ISBN-13: 978-1475152180

DEDICATION

First and foremost, this book is dedicated to my husband who always wanted me to publish although my guess is he did not envision this as the topic for my first book. It is also dedicated to those who share this journey with me, the unsung heroes and heroines who manage from day to day and who make life changing decisions as caregivers and still somehow hold on to their own inner self.

CONTENTS

Acknowledgements (i)
Introduction (1)
Lost on a Civilized Island (2)
Seeing the Light in the Fog (3)
Short Course in Grieving & Therapy (4)
When I Became Legion (6)
Home Coming to Someone Else's Home (7)
The Path to Mental Breakdown (10)
Adjusting After the Island (18)
The Visit (20)
Another Major Change – "We" Must Leave (21)
The Trail Back (23)
Finding a New "Normal" (27)
Show & Tell & Tolkien Languages (30)
Prodigal Pronouns (33)
Time is an Essence (34)
Stealing Mail (38)
The Magic Desk & Other Disappearing Acts (39)
Fixing the Coffee Pot (40)
Buying Clothes & Other Closet Adventures (42)
Personal Hygiene & Other Cleaning Guides (46)
Medical Issues & Playing Nurse (50)
Books & Magazines (57)
Movies & TV Shows (59)
Through Thick & Thin & Emily Post (61)
Grocery Shopping & Anything Goes (65)
Telephones That Translate & Other Tele-tales (68)
Ears & Other Removable Parts (71)
Unlearning to Drive (74)
Finances in Fantasy Land (76)
Legally Speaking (81)
Relationships with Real & "Real" People (84)
Becoming Who I Am to Him (90)

ACKNOWLEDGMENTS

First, I must acknowledge the friends and relatives who convinced me that my story should be heard. I also must thank a very dear and precious friend who volunteered to be my editor. I know her to have unflinching grammatical standards and if I missed any of her corrections the fault is mine. A second reading was provided with the help of a Facebook friend. I also want to acknowledge a publisher that let me do it my way.

As an added note, there are a few quotes in this little book from the Desiderata. This beautiful piece of prose was not nailed to the door of St. Paul's Church in Baltimore, nor is it all that old. It was written by Max Ehrmann in the 1920s. In 1976 the 7th Circuit Court of Appeals ruled that the copyright had been forfeited since it had been published freely since 1940 without copyright notice. Therefore, the piece was declared public domain. Mr. Ehrmann's family had received a few royalties from earlier publications. I believe Mr. Ehrmann deserves credit for a succinct statement of "desired things." It is an inspiration and well worth looking up in full for:

"You are a child of the universe
no less than the trees and the stars;
you have a right to be here.
And whether or not it is clear to you,
no doubt the universe is unfolding as it should."

Remember that as you walk with me on this journey....

Introduction

Months after the events described here started, a friend of mine posted a rather interesting poster on Facebook which seemed to wrap up my life in a neat little cliché. The picture was a sign that said: "I'm lost. I've gone to look for myself. If I should return before I get back, please ask me to wait." This became my life, the reality I dealt with each and every day. And this is the story of how I learned to cope. Or, at least how I survived the first shock wave of losing the man I love, my best friend, the first person in the world I learned to really trust. It is also a story about learning something of how the human mind works, of the depths of feeling two people can have for each other and how precious a thing our lives together can be.

No, this companion, my soul mate and husband didn't die; his mind did, inch by inch. All my life, after the initial shock and emotional reaction of a situation, I have worked my way through "the next step" in a carefully thought out, logical sequence. Sometimes the resolution to the current problem was quick; sometimes it took a great deal of planning and patience. This new challenge will take me years of working and re-working "the plan." Perhaps in the sharing of my struggle, I will learn about me and him, and maybe help others do the same for themselves.

I fell in love with this man knowing that our age difference may someday require that I become a caregiver. I accepted that reality and, even now, would not forgo our years together simply to avoid the heartbreak I now sometimes experience. And, when he thanks me for the simplest things I do for him, or reaches out to touch me in the night, or seems so happy when I call during the day, I feel a special kind of quiet joy that I still mean that much to him; Whoever I Am Yesterday. This, then, is our story.

Lost on a Civilized Island

Although there were signs for many months, perhaps even years; signs that I saw but didn't see, arguments about what I did or did not tell him, or what he did or did not control in his life, there was a day, an hour, a moment when I could no longer blame the problems on any other source. We had planned for several months to take a vacation to Vancouver Island, British Columbia. We had saved for it, gone over travel brochures, worked with a travel agent and researched places to see and stay. I was even going to try for a job interview or two to see what the possibility was of us moving to a warmer climate and a place nearer the sea.

The morning we got up to catch the plane things were suddenly very strange. At first I thought it was the hour, after all 4:00 in the morning was pretty early. He told me he thought the people who were taking us to the airport had forgotten us. I told him no, we were right on time, but that we should hurry in order to be sure we had the time we needed. We drove to the airport, parked the car in long term parking and caught a shuttle to the terminal. We sat and had coffee before going to the gate and talked about nothing much in particular. Our conversation seemed to be normal, or maybe I was just excited that we were finally going to visit a place we had talked so much about for months, if not years. Now that we were finally going I didn't want to see anything that might prevent us. As we sat in the gate area waiting for the plane he asked me who had paid me to go with him. Say, what?

He seemed fairly normal during the flight. We watched the plane travel across the Rockies on the graphic in front of our seats and looked out the window at the snow covered peaks below us. He read a little from his magazines. He seemed happy, but somewhat subdued.

After we landed I was pretty intent on trying to get organized. I had actually forgotten what name I had reserved the car under and there was a bit of panic until I was able to confirm the reservation; which I had actually made in his name.

He stood patiently, guarding our luggage, while I sorted things out. I remember being concerned about leaving him alone for very long, as if he might disappear. Once things were settled, we walked through the drizzle at the Victoria airport, found the car and started out.

Although I had been somewhat nervous about the responses I had been receiving from him that morning, I was even more concerned when his initial line of questioning did not stop. Suddenly I had changed from being his wife to being his business and travel companion from many years before. Or, at least it seemed so. At first I really thought he was teasing me, but no, he really did think I was someone from his past. Our years together had suddenly vanished. Lost, in the middle of a beautiful island, the vacation I had so looked forward to became my boot camp for living with vascular dementia.

Seeing the Light in the Fog

Our week on the Island was a step by step course in elementary attitude adjustment. Our drive from Victoria to Nanaimo was drippy and foggy and every bit the type of atmosphere expected in the great Northwest. During that drive I pieced together a number of important things that I had to grasp in order to care for my husband in the future. He really did not remember being married to me. He insisted it had been a very long time since he had seen me and that he was sorry he had left me. Frustrated, I tried to explain that we were married, that we had lived together for a number of years, and that we lived together in Calgary. No, no. It was that "other woman" that lived there, not me.

As we drove up the coast and stopped for lunch, I kept pressing. Desperate, I looked for any link that would remind him, any correlation that would reach him; and nothing did. Slowly I realized that I was only making him angry, driving him further away from me. In some ways he had already left me, I didn't want to push him so far that I wasn't even a dream from the past. Thus, the first light: the world in his eyes would never be the same and would change with every day. If I wanted to keep him, I would have to move through those worlds with him and not try to keep him in mine.

Short Course In Grieving & Therapy

There were times when things seemed almost normal. Then he would jolt me with questions about who was paying for all of this. He would ask when he was going to meet the people he came to see, or, how was he going to get home? The concept of things being paid for with "our" money was just not acceptable to him. He felt he needed to reimburse me for what I was spending. He emptied his pockets of all his cash and gave it to me, "just to help." We had planned to meet someone regarding his research work, but I just couldn't bring myself to make any calls when I was never sure where his conversation would lead. And, again, the repeated theme of asking how he was going to get back to the house where he lived and where all his books were kept.

During a quick trip to the store our second day there, I called our doctor who suggested I get him to a clinic and check for a urinary tract infection. There was one and we treated it: it wasn't enough. Whether it was a combination of the infection, the plane trip or it was just time, my husband had disappeared somewhere within his mind never to return. Consequently, I became determined to make that trip the vacation of our lives.

From our base in Nanaimo we visited local beaches often. We drove to Qualicum Bay and Parksville. One day we drove up into the mountains west of Nanaimo and visited a state park. Another day we drove to Port Alberni, stopping to spend time in the Cathedral Grove and walking on the shores of Sproat Lake. Another day we drove to Tofino and walked the Pacific Rim Trail in Ucluelet. We also visited the downtown area of Nanaimo to look at the marina and ferry docks. All along the way I took every opportunity to walk with him, talk, hold hands, and let him be whatever he wanted or needed to be. We even purchased souvenirs, something I usually avoid.

Our conversations were occasionally about perfectly normal subjects, sometimes meaningless meandering I simply could not follow. I took pictures everywhere we went. Months later while we were looking at the photos in my computer with some friends he asked if he could have copies. Those photos (all 225 of them) are now in an album he keeps in his office. I'm not really sure what they mean to him, but I hold on to the knowledge that they mean something.

In a moment alone, after one of those interviews I did manage to make, I called a friend of mine. She is someone who knows home health care, geriatrics, and just what care giving is all about. The first words out of my mouth were, "I'm losing him." The strain in my voice must have been evident because she asked what hospital he was in. While I barely held onto my emotions we talked about what sort of options I might have. I told her the doctor had said he would be in a home within the year. Her response was, "No he won't. You will need help but I know you, you can handle it." So began my thought process. What plans do I make, what changes must happen, and how long do I have to make them?

In another moment alone, while he wandered on a beach within sight, I also called his eldest son. It had been my hope that I could reach him before his father was too mentally weakened. I wanted him to have some time with his Dad that could be remembered. (You see, I did know what was happening). In tears, I apologized for possibly waiting too long. Of all the people who have supported me during this change, I have to say my stepson has been one of the most precious. Although I had never been close to his family (in fact, I had only met him once) he was very supportive and encouraged me to share what was going on in our lives. He would drop a quick email and ask for a report about what things were going well and what things were not so great. He took time away from his own family to visit us for a week a few months after our return. I'll return to that later. All in all he helped to keep the lonely, isolated feelings at bay.

While still on the Island I contacted my employer and extended my vacation an extra day. I needed time to make contacts, watch him at home back in his own territory, and to start to weave together the pieces necessary for our new life together. It also gave me one more day to cry the tears that he could not see: he would not have understood. The timing of our trip was nothing short of miraculous. I really don't know how I would have worked through the initial shock if it had been necessary to go to work each day not knowing what I would find when I returned. Not knowing how much time I needed to take off for us both to adjust. Or even trying to learn to cope without the calming affects of trees and mountains, lakes and seas. I suddenly knew how starved I was for the nature I love so much. My refuge. My own special therapy.

When I Became Legion

As mentioned, we were staying in Nanaimo and had arrived late in the afternoon of our first day. Our room had a tiny kitchen corner so that we could save on meal costs during our stay and was pretty centrally located for all the places we had planned to see. The weather for the rest of the week was absolutely beautiful. He seemed comfortable being with me no matter where we went, after all, I was his long lost girlfriend. At least at the moment. Ever watchful, I tried to learn to answer his questions with patience as if he had never been told before. Where were my parents? Did I have siblings? Where did I live? One night he woke up and asked whose stuff was hanging in the corner? He would stand by the shores of lakes and the Georgia Strait and tell me all about what "they" wanted him to do, in terms I no longer understood. Then he would ask me about the lady that was with him yesterday.

He had remembered that we were supposed to contact someone about his work and wondered when we would see them: then he told me they had called. He saw them; people had come to talk to him. Didn't I know these people? He was sure they were part of "my team." Each day was a test. The odd thing is that I always seem to be "me" at the present moment (not his wife, just me), but even now I am never sure of Who I Am Yesterday, or even a few hours ago.

So I spent our vacation week learning, testing, watching, and hoping. But it was also a week of spending time with my beloved in the most beautiful place we had been for a long, long time. We managed to wander through that emotional minefield and actually, I believe, enjoy ourselves. Yes, I cried. Buckets. Quiet, private, buckets.

When I did leave for brief periods for those job interviews he seemed fine when I returned. I was the one that had trouble figuring out who left and who came back. I kept hoping, though, that once I got him home something would trigger his memory. Something, anything would reach him and he might understand something of what was happening. I kept telling him I could show him these things he did not believe once we returned to Calgary. "I have pictures, I have documents, and there are people that know us. Just wait, I'll show you." I asked him to be patient and reassured him that we had plane tickets and that we were scheduled to return. And yes, I knew he had lots of books, no really, *lots* of books.

Our week in a far away land came to an end, and so it was, as I had promised him, that I took him back to Calgary where all his things were kept.

Home Coming to Someone Else's Home

When we arrived at the Victoria airport we were rather early. The airlines put us on an earlier flight, which would give me more time at "home" to try to get oriented. We got off the plane and caught the shuttle to long term parking. I showed him that we both had keys to the same car and that I knew what that car was like and where it was parked. As we drove to the house he said it looked like I might be taking him home and was surprised we weren't going to "my house" first. Arriving at the house I showed him I had keys to doors, garage door openers, and knowledge of where things were. All of that did not matter. He was worried that "she" might be there. Didn't I have somewhere else to stay? Really, was there nowhere else I could sleep; not even my mother's house? As it happens my mother lived 350 miles away in another country. Suddenly, I was homeless. My whole life was in that house and, suddenly, it wasn't mine anymore. It belonged to some woman that he didn't think he wanted anymore. I kept thinking he was confusing me with some other woman in his life. It was days before I realized that woman was some version of me.

Getting resettled was an experience. He didn't know what we would do with all "her" stuff. Shouldn't we throw out "her" clothes? Did I really want to read "her" books? I should be made aware that some of those books were his and not "hers." If I really didn't have anywhere else to go, did I want to stay with him? He was very nice about it all, running around trying to show me where things were, letting me know where things were kept and what worked and what didn't. In fact, it seemed to be a bit of a race to see if he could show me before I simply picked up a bowl or pot or towel, or walked into a room to retrieve something we needed.

I turned on the computer and asked him to look at our wedding pictures. He agreed it looked like him and was sorry if I had been mislead; but that wasn't him. I showed him our marriage certificate; that wasn't his signature. Just because our rings matched was no indication that we had been married: "she" wore one just like it. He mentioned he might have to explain who I was to the next door neighbor. Through the tears I wondered how that would turn out. I told him I knew them and he wasn't sure he believed me. Finally, I called the couple who had known us almost as long as we had been in Canada; in fact, they were the witnesses at our wedding. They, in their ever-loving way, dropped everything to come and see us the next day.

When they came in the door I, quite frankly, collapsed in their arms. He seemed surprised that I should know them. His comment was "I guess I don't have to introduce you." I still don't understand why he had no problem recognizing our neighbors or our friends, the way home from the airport, our house; but didn't "see" me. They spent the better part of the morning with us trying to soften the blow. He told them that he liked me and that he didn't mind staying with me, but he didn't know where "she" had gone. They did their best to prepare me to be comfortable being whatever woman it was he thought I was at the moment. That afternoon he wanted me to change the locks so "she" couldn't get back in. No, I didn't, and he eventually let it drop.

There was a time for the first week or so when something in his mind said: "this is not making sense." Somewhere the logic that had driven his research career for over five decades was kicking in and saying, "Wait, this does not add up." I thought I had a window of opportunity and as he asked me those penetrating questions I used the things he could remember to build a case that he wasn't thinking quite like he should. He spent some time thinking about all that we discussed, and for a day or so I thought maybe…maybe he will at least accept that something is happening and we can go from there. That moment passed. There was no amount of information, talking or badgering that would bring him to realize that something was very, very wrong.

There was one evening when I returned home to find that he was certain he was dying. Even then, as I listened to what he said, to his sense of urgency to do what he felt he must do, I didn't think he meant physically. I believe he knew he was slipping away mentally and did not know what to do about it. He still had ideas he wanted to explore, concepts he wanted to get on paper, and he was losing his grasp. I have found through the months of our "adventure" that if I want to work with him, keep him healthy, happy, and cooperative, mentioning his mental condition is out of the question. I am forever thankful that I found medical professionals that understood that and worked with me to achieve the best healthcare he could have without his full and unconditional cooperation. Recently I watched as a specialist carefully explained to him that the condition we were discussing would not impact his ability to fly a plane. Well, it doesn't.

The Path to Mental Breakdown

Perhaps someday it will be worthwhile to put our whole story on paper. I feel it is important to provide some background so that his mental state is seen in context. I met my husband in April of 1994. He was introduced by mutual friends and was in the last stages of a divorce. I, at the time, was married. No, it was not a happy marriage and I was in the process of becoming rather alienated from the world around me. This man jolted me out of that attitude overnight. He was brilliant (really, his publication record proves that). I could listen to his voice for hours; we talked for hours. We talked about philosophy, religion, mathematics, political science, literature and a whole host of other things. We didn't always agree, but we could always discuss. It was nearly two years before we found ourselves in a situation that brought us together on a personal and intimate level.

For a number of years we worked together to form a company that would market and develop his research. The only problem was that we started our search for funds at the crest of the dot.com era. No amount of marketing skills could convince an investor that this was *not* the type of "technology company" that was crashing and burning on every side. In the fall of 2001, my marriage over, I sold everything I could and moved to Washington to be with him.

I suppose I should have noticed things even then. I was drawn into a dream that the two of us had created. Having spent large portions of my life dealing with stalkers, his paranoia did not strike me as strange. In fact, my innate sense of always watching my back probably helped to draw him to me in the first place. However, during our entire five years in Washington (he was not always living with me) I do not believe he was actually employed. According to him, he was always involved in something with the government. Something which

I was told involved his research, his inability to get compensated for the things he had done, or his need to defend his ownership of his work.

Before that chuckle in your mind breaks out into laughter, you should recall that this was a period of time when there were documented cases of people who had developed software and had somehow lost control of the copyright as it suddenly became government property. We had stories of newspaper people threatened with treason, undercover agents being exposed, and a government that couldn't seem to think up enough ways to gain more and more control of its citizens. His story was not that fantastic in that context. He had a strong publication record and piles of technical papers he had contributed to in the defense industry. He also had evidence of a past security clearance. This was no ordinary man. There was just enough hard evidence to make his claims plausible.

At some point his concerns of persecution reached a critical point; at least for me. I found a way to remove us from the people he was so afraid of and travel to Canada. Two months before leaving Washington he experienced a seizure. Evidently he had experienced a seizure some twenty years earlier. He had taken the prescribed medication for six months, and he had been weaned off of it never to experience another issue until the fall of 2006. The doctors put him back on anti-convulsants. During our last few months in Washington I watched him carefully. Our plans were already in motion and he didn't seem inclined to change them.

As the packing came close to the deadline he seemed to become quite frustrated. The task seemed overwhelming for him and I ended up taking care of a number of things to keep it all in motion. November 30, 2006 we started our trek to Canada in our two cars. And, yes, he believed we were in peril, and consequently so did I. Months later I spoke with one of our neighbors who informed me that someone had come to the door looking for us and saying she was my sister. My sister knew how to find me if need be and had no reason to be in Washington. These are the types of things that haunted us.

The first leg of our journey was rather uneventful. We had planned to stop in Plains, Montana to relieve ourselves of a few more assets, set up addresses and bank accounts in case anyone was looking for us and to see my mother and a few close friends. While we were there he experienced another seizure. We later determined it was most likely because he had missed a dose of his medication. There is a good chance he simply forgot since he was trying to nurse me back to health from a rather nasty cold and a wicked migraine. At some point during that seizure, or in the aftermath, he suffered a compression fracture in his knee. So much for driving: let alone a standard shift. Switching from two cars to one, and starting off with an articulating cast to avoid surgery, we completed our journey to Calgary, Alberta.

The details of our experience in Canada will have to be saved for some other time, perhaps the aforementioned story of our lives. Suffice it to say that as soon as we could legally work I began to try to find ways and means of marketing his research. While, of course, I worked a job that would pay our bills and help us reduce our enormous debt. It seemed to me that he did not pursue these things himself; he relied on me greatly to find resources, communicate his background and even set up meetings.

Due to the fracture and the seizures I have to admit I became rather protective. There were many things that he simply could not do while he was in the cast and I became his temporary caregiver. Even after his recovery, it was some time before I could get him back behind the wheel of a car. Always, though, when we were with someone who could understand; and I could get him started, his mind would click in gear and he would be in that place where he truly lived. He had no problem discussing pattern recognition, explaining concepts of artificial intelligence or finding appropriate papers that he had authored to explain his points. He had, however, lost the ability to handle the social side of marketing one's skills. I chose to not internalize that difference: I covered for it.

Sometime after we moved into the home we occupied for over four years the "people" started showing up again. I was never certain if they were good guys or bad guys; there seemed to be some of both. I asked him to take pictures but there was always some excuse. I would look for footprints in the snow; sometimes there were some. He would tell me about little boys looking in the windows down stairs, when, quite frankly, those windows were under decks or cantilevered windows. He eventually covered the windows up. It would have been extremely difficult in earlier years to determine how much of his paranoia had a basis in reality: now it is impossible.

During the past year I have read a book entitled, *The Believing Brain*, by Michael Shermer. There was much in this book I found of interest. Most importantly, Dr. Shermer provides a supportable explanation as to why genius and madness dance so closely together in the human mind. The reason brilliant people develop and dream of the most amazing things is because they see patterns where the majority of people do not. The down side is that they are even more susceptible to seeing patterns where none exist. Thus, while my husband could envision many truly brilliant applications for mathematics and physics, he also saw things that were nothing more than a construct of his own mind.

Something in him knew this challenge because when I would try to get him to introduce me to some of these "visitors" the anger would come. It would be better if he left, he didn't want me in danger, and he should find a way to be somewhere else. And I would fight back. You can't leave me. I really don't know what I would do without you, and (to myself) I don't know how you would survive without me. I handled all of our finances, making sure that his Social Security and pension serviced his enormous credit card debt while my salary paid the rent, utilities and food bill (and my slightly less enormous debt). I quite honestly knew he couldn't make it alone.

Yet, he functioned as most any other person would in our little world. He spoke with our attorney in clear terms of what he did or did not want. Meaning, he volunteered specific clauses he wanted in Personal Directives and wills. He even suggested who we should use as an agent on the paperwork and made sure we contacted his eldest son to convey that preference. He helped me, without request, around the house. We read and visited places near our home. We visited with our closest friends, and we talked about all those things we had always loved to talk about. And, somehow, I allowed myself to slip into survival mode. Waiting on the Canadian government to make a decision on our application for residency, going to work each day to earn a living, and coming home to deal with our personal issues and handle a few contract clients. Even still trying to find someone somewhere who would be interested in taking the piles of research in our basement and compiling them into something useful if not completely lucrative. Then the world began to spiral out of control.

It was a morning like any other bone-chilling morning in January in Calgary. I drove off to work arriving somewhere between 6:30 and 7:00 and, as was my habit, started to call the house to let him know I had safely arrived. He didn't answer. For an hour I could not reach him. Finally I called our next door neighbor, scared to death he had fallen on the slick driveway and was freezing to death in the cold. Quite possible since it was somewhere around 30 below Celsius. The neighbor said she would be happy to check on him and would call me back. She could see lights on in the house, so he probably had not gone back to bed.

Frantic, I continued to call until I finally reached her at our kitchen table. He had fallen. She didn't say where at that time but she did say he had a rather bad bump on his head and she and her husband would be taking him to the hospital. One of my co-workers asked if I needed help (without my car near me I would have accepted), another offered to explain what was happening to my supervisor. I ran back to my car parked four blocks away and forced myself to stop for gas not knowing what I would have to deal with the rest of the day. I tried to call my neighbors' house and their daughter answered saying they had already left. I asked if he had fallen outside. She didn't know. She only knew her mother came back to the house screaming for her father and saying my husband had "cracked his skull open." Wow, that was reassuring. I met them at the hospital just as he was going through triage.

Bump, cracked skull? What he had done was a pretty good job of trying to scalp himself. The best our friends and I were ever able to put together is that he had fallen backwards into the pony wall on our stairwell and the corner of the wall had sliced open his scalp. Evidently when my poor neighbor had talked him into opening the door (he was rather dazed at the time) he had blood all over his face. She cleaned things up a bit before taking him off to emergency. The gash was rather nasty. I was at his side all day leaving only to call his eldest son and my supervisor with updates. I was with him when the nurse and the doctor put in the five stitches and fifteen staples.

The doctors and I were never able to determine if he suffered another seizure or just tripped. What did happen is a lot of confusion in his mind about how he got those staples. I blamed it on the concussion. The doctor in emergency was able to confirm there was no fracture, but it takes a rather severe "bump" to open up a gash maybe an inch wide on one end and, perhaps, four inches long. Even though I told him I was there when he got those staples, he still didn't seem to believe me. It also, sadly, put some sort of barrier in his mind against that incredible neighbor lady. He never seemed to trust her after that. My only guess is that she saw him in a very vulnerable situation and he could not handle that kind of situation with another person; in the end, not even me. After all, I wasn't there that day helping to clean his wound, rubbing his feet while they put in the stitches and the staples, or giving him water with a sponge while he was still in the neck collar.

Even the friendship he had with the gentleman next door suffered. This supportive friend and neighbor stayed with him while I ran to the store that night. Like me, he had trouble keeping him down so the bleeding wouldn't start again. Apparently, my husband thought he should be carrying groceries, helping with setting the table and helping with dinner. Our neighbor brought one of his carpet cleaners to the house and cleaned up the blood on the carpet where my husband had fallen. My husband avoided the spot entirely, never actually looking at what was going on although he usually watched everything our neighbor did. Our neighbor also kept a close eye on him when I returned to work a week later. But all that only made my husband more protective. He was sure that the man was interested in me. Of course, according to him, all men are interested in me, and that's OK, what in the world would I want with him?

That was January 2011. Due to the fall the doctor scheduled several tests to see if there were any problems we needed to be aware of. There were MRI's, EEG's, scans, and visits with a neurologist. He was so uncomfortable with the MRI and EEG that I had to be with him while the tests were conducted. The EEG technician commented that there was quite a lot of activity and things looked rather well. The MRI technician was only able to get one set of scans. Neither the technician or myself could get him to stay on the table. Somehow I believe he knew what was wrong and didn't really want to know for sure, or for anyone else to guess. His whole attitude changed from grouchy and uncooperative to cheery and talkative the moment we started to walk out of the hospital.

What we got, however, was enough to produce a diagnosis of vascular dementia. At the neurological clinic we spent several hours with tests and interviews. It was evident to me that his memory and his abilities had suffered a serious blow. He could not recognize certain animals, draw a clock or count backwards. He swore up and down he did not have a memory problem: I knew he did. The medical record indicates that I agreed with his protestations; an unfair assessment since I was being asked in his presence. What I did say to him was, "dear, everyone forgets something sometime." "No, not me," he responds: "Never."

Afterwards he seemed to come back to some form of "normal." Perhaps he was slower and in need of more repetition. In fact I expanded on my little journals of what we had to do and what had been done. I always typed up important events, doctor's visits, what doctors said; things we needed to do, and gave him a copy. When I spoke with our clinic's psychologist some time later, she asked me if that was time consuming. I told her it couldn't be any more time consuming than repeating oneself over and over every day. Or trying to figure out if I was the one losing it because I was almost certain I had told him something he insisted I had not. That one hour with her gave me the steam to keep going a few more months. All along, we still did dishes together, he still did his laundry, he still wrote while I was away during the day. And I still clung to my remaining pieces of denial. I had called the psychologist because I was frustrated in my job, I had just been told that my husband did, indeed have dementia, and I had no idea how I was going to handle my fracturing world and avoid falling into the dark hole of my own bi-polar brain. She gave me light.

Perhaps it would be helpful to mention that I rarely talk to other people about what is going on in my life. At least it had not been my habit to share my feelings, hurts and disappointments. Not until this man entered my life. He really was my best friend. He listened and provided advice. Not always advice that I took, but always with insight that gave me options so I could make my own choices. That late winter day when the doctor told me that the results did indeed indicate dementia I was suddenly alone again. There was no one to talk to. No one to discuss what I should or should not do with my job. No one to tell me how to care for my best friend and partner. This is why I sought out our clinic's psychologist.

I had spoken with her once before during our intake to the clinic. This I did because I was and am an un-medicated bi-polar. My husband was a very good watcher and under different circumstances he could have been my alarm system for when it was time to accept help. Help sought based on his advice I would have been prepared to accept. It seemed prudent to let our medical team know of the background so they, too, could spot issues. Now, my beacon was gone and I was alone. This wonderful professional helped me get my feet back under me and helped me focus on our future rather than my fears.

Even now I do not attend a support group, but that is my choice based on my life experiences. One day I may find that I must make the time to meet with others in my own situation. Since those first desperate months, I have found that I do have dear friends, more than I ever knew, who support me and give me strength at some of my darkest moments. One very dear friend, who knows us both well, reassured me in a moment of despair and discovery that whatever the source of my husband's mental failure was; he and I were meant for each other. There was no doubt in our friend's mind that if the situation had been reversed my husband would have been at my side working out some way to protect our future. This friend is not known as a romantic individual, but he has always been supportive during this journey through wonder-land. And, for now, talking to you here at my computer is really the best therapy for me. If you need help to find balance; find it. You will do no one any good, least of all yourself, if you try to "brave it through" and lose yourself in the process.

Adjusting After the Island

So, here we were living in a home that wasn't home, in a marriage that didn't happen, with ghosts in the closet (if not in every corner) and the need to survive. I started to realize why he didn't like "that other woman" very much. She was gone most of the waking hours, worked every weekend, never seemed to go anywhere and caused all sorts of problems when she seemed to doubt his version of things. Oh, and she would read in bed at night. "That woman" had become his jailor.

I, on the other hand, was another story. He asked me if I liked reading in the evening and having wine while I was in the jet tub (you know this is "her" wine, it's OK if you have it). He asked me questions about my family (many, many times) and my "team" grew. He found it interesting that I worked at the same place as "she" did, liked the same things, wore the same clothes, and yet: "she" was gone. Late one afternoon he told me he didn't understand why she would leave and not say anything. Didn't I know how to get in touch with her? Was she OK? The only response that I could come up with is that she never would have left him willingly and I believed she was doing as well as could be expected. At least that was the truth, if nothing else was.

I also started making changes in our life. I purchased a TV and a DVD player. Although he never learned to use the remotes, he did enjoy most evenings watching a movie or a show. We had watched movies on my computer on the weekends, but I extended that in hopes of providing outside stimulation. We loved watching the nature programs (for awhile) and there was a time when he let me watch M*A*S*H; until that became a problem for some inexplicable reason. Picking things he would like could be a minefield. The most success I have had is stories about music and dancing and romantic comedies: not sure how that happened. If the concepts were abstract and not simple boy-girl or happy ending; then he just couldn't follow it.

I also changed my work hours so I could come home an hour earlier. He could not understand why those people made me stay so long. Explaining to him that "they" paid me to work for 40 hours (or more) a week made no sense to him. He was sure "they" were taking advantage of me. When I would try to explain that we needed the money to pay the rent, buy groceries, keep the house warm; well, he just couldn't make sense of it. Why did we have to pay rent? Could he help with the groceries? I had accumulated a pile of overtime and I used it to spend more time at home with him. I also turned up the heat on looking for a new job on the coast and near the water he loved so much. And I started working on a way to bring my work home on a contractual basis. There were a few days I wasn't sure *that* would work. As I'll explain later, dementia steals the concept of time. Everything is in the moment and if it can't be done now there is no other time.

There was a co-worker at my office, a sensitive person that did pick up on my various phone calls. Over a year earlier she had caught pieces of conversations I was having trying to get care for my mother who was in serious condition. This time she again came to my side and offered a shoulder. She had recently lost a sister to cancer and understood some of what I was going through. The difference, of course, was that when I went home my loss was still there, but not there; taunting me with what would never be. She helped me step through that phase and to move on in the journey of grief so that I could build a future and not bury myself in the land of "might have been." She also encouraged me to talk with our human resources department to explore options that might help me handle the situation.

Slowly I started to create a different atmosphere in which we could live. I reassured him I was looking for alternatives to life in Calgary; in the cold and much too far from the beaches he so loved. That July his son came to visit. His son and I had arranged it in the background and when he spoke to his father on Father's Day he announced his plans. My husband was confused as to why his son should suddenly want to visit; I brushed off those questions by indicating it had been a long time and with his grandchildren growing up, perhaps his son wanted to reconnect with his own father. Well, that was better than saying he wants to see you before you no longer recognize him!

The Visit

As it turned out his father had no problem recognizing him, and it is my hope that some benefit came from the time they had together. Even though his son had to work while he was with us, we had pleasant evenings together. That was probably the last time that my husband fixed something to eat on his own. It was only a tuna sandwich, but he never managed even that much again.

I am told that they did have nice conversations from time to time. His son told me that they would be talking along about something and suddenly the subject would change and things would become jumbled. He tried to get some sense of what his father had been researching to let me know if I should do something with his things; but all those doors were always locked. Physically and mentally. Evidently trust did not extend to his own son. Only I was honored with the second set of keys, whoever I was that day.

I had asked his son what he remembered best about his childhood. He told me he liked the times the family had gone hiking, skiing or fishing. So, I planned a trip to Elbow Falls west of Calgary and we spent a lovely late afternoon walking up and down the park's trails. My husband and I were treated to a great dinner in the little town of Bragg Creek. When we returned home I truly felt it was time well spent for all of us. We took our visitor back to the airport the next morning.

Later, I put together a small picture album of the whole week and sent it to my stepson. It still gives me some bittersweet memories to browse through the short pages. For many months afterward my dear husband would make comments about the visit, even if the reference points were a bit off. Best of all, during the visit he even mentioned our anniversary. We went out on that night and it is probably the last time he was in agreement regarding our state of matrimony. July 12, 2011.

Another Major Change – "We" Must Leave

It was in December of that year that the Canadian government let us know that they did not want us as permanent residents. We received the decision nearly five years to the day from when we had entered the country. Although the agent could not provide a firm date, we had, at most, six weeks to plan our move back to the United States.

This is not the place to go into the fears I faced and conquered. Things about economies, employment, money to move, and how long we would actually be allowed to execute the move. As it happened, because I had taken concrete steps to leave the country, the border agent assigned to our case was willing to work on my time schedule. It was still quite a task.

Packing was the first issue. Since we had some 16,420 pounds of things (actual weight from the manifest) the majority of which was books and files, we started packing during the Christmas holidays. Funny, that isn't exactly what I had in mind when I scheduled that week off! At first my husband was overwhelmed with the task, but as things progressed he actually contributed quite a bit to the packing of his library.

I wasn't certain what his feelings were about the move. I know that he was tired of being cooped up and really did not like the dry cold of Calgary. He made some references to the people in the United States that could harm him, but it wasn't the desperate sort of thing that I would have seen only a year or two before. He did say he wanted to see the people "where the waters are" that had talked to him. I told him I was taking him to Seattle and he would be closer to them and could communicate with them when we arrived. Sometime between Vancouver Island and Seattle he decided that the government wanted him to go on a mission in space. Since he had done some work for NASA, this wasn't entirely off the charts. Sometimes I felt like I wouldn't mind going with him.

Finding a job was a priority until the manager where I worked told me that they would keep me on as a contract/virtual manager during and after the move. Documents were drawn up that would protect my position for at least another 60 days. What a miracle to have this bridge to get us to our new home and put me in a position to look for additional work while I still had income. The company eventually extended that contract well into summer and my career as a consultant was launched. I only needed to hold on to it.

The Trail Back

    Several things were involved in the planning of our move. We had, of course, been hoping for a move to Vancouver Island, not Seattle. While we were planning that approach, our neighbor had mentioned that he would be willing to drive a truck. At first my husband wanted me to know that his neighbor had promised to move all the books. Somehow a moving truck and our neighbor's motor home got confused in his mind and he was certain that it was that big bus that was going to move us. Then something happened I have yet to understand and he didn't want the neighbor helping us at all. He wanted to control our things, after all he could drive that truck (no, please no).

    When our neighbor could no longer commit, I tried the approach of having friends from the United States drive a truck if I paid the expenses. When I had a local moving company come out to quote packing the truck that all went to pieces. The man informed me that he thought the largest truck I could rent was about 6 feet short and would be seriously short on the weight allowance. Oops. As it happens the largest private rental was only rated at about half of our total load. Thus, we had to find a commercial mover and the lowest possible rate I could negotiate. Meantime, the clock was ticking. I called the people who had moved our things north nearly five years before and cut a fast and tight deal.

    Knowing we would have to take our time, neither one of us could take the long, long hours behind the wheel anymore, I planned several days to get from Calgary to Seattle through Plains, Montana. Hotel rates in Plains are much lower than in Seattle so a couple of days catching up with banking, relatives and friends would be an solid economic choice. The truck, however, would follow a shorter route and meet us in Seattle. We had the help of a friend, that same home caregiver, to find a suitable rental so we had an endpoint to go to. Trying to arrive in Seattle and store things or find a home while the truck was on the road didn't seem practical. So, I paid the rent for the month to hold the house even though we wouldn't be there until sometime around the tenth.

While the truck was being loaded, the driver, a day late because of a delay at the border, happened to mention he would see me in a couple of weeks. Not having a lot of capacity for changes at that moment, and knowing I was already paying rent on a house we weren't living in, I immediately contacted the moving company and asked them if they had any concept of the word "contract." Moves can be unpredictable and moving companies cannot control weather or border agencies, but to be so cavalier as to assume that the driver could mosey on down to Seattle whenever he had some personal things taken care of; well, I probably wasn't very nice. I was told by our booking agent that he would get it all sorted out and not to worry. He did push them to deliver on time, even if they chose the outside date I had contracted for.

All the while I kept working on my job on a borrowed laptop, right up until the moment they loaded my desk. When it was all said and done and we had said our goodbyes to the landlord, handed over the keys and provided contact information, we headed for a hotel near the highway so we could get a reasonably early start. Before sleeping I geared up the laptop and kept on working.

The next day was to be our longest day on the road in more ways than one. My husband did not want to stop for lunch; he wanted to know where we were going. Did I know where we were going? Shouldn't I catch up to the car in front of us and ask where we were going? When were we going to get there? I should drive faster so we could talk to that person and find out where we were.

Finally, after what seemed to be days, we arrived in Kalispell and stopped at the first reasonably good looking restaurant to have dinner. He kept asking if I knew the place (no), how did I find it (looking), how much further (about 90 minutes or so). He recognized nothing. Not the lake we had spent so many pleasant (and passionate) days and nights at, not the town he had lived in, visited, and purchased property in.

The hopes I had that were growing ever thinner were dashed the following morning when he still did not recognize a single thing in the town where he had spent so much time and where he had planned to retire. Absolutely nothing seemed to spark a sense of recognition in him. We, in fact, stayed in the very same room we had stayed in when passing through the town a bit over five years before. Not even a glimmer.

For months he had wanted to meet my mother and I had thought he just might recognize her when he did. No, not even vaguely. I had to work from her house the day we were there due to issues with wireless connections on the laptop. I left him in her care in the front room while I tried to catch up on my workload. She said that there were times when he could discuss the varied subjects they both had interest in without missing a beat: then the subject would suddenly change and nothing would be connected. He later told me she seemed sad and felt she had nothing left to do. Not a vision I really had of my mother. She is a survivor like her mother before her or she wouldn't have been sitting there talking to him. Perhaps the sadness was his own. The next morning we started the next leg of our journey.

He didn't seem quite as anxious on the drive from Plains to Moses Lake, Washington. I think, in part, because we were not out in the middle of nowhere with no one in sight for hours and hours as we had been on the drive from Calgary. And, I made sure we were not in the car as long. He still wanted to know where we were going and I had to keep reassuring him that we had a place to stay in Seattle and he could make contact with the people he needed to talk to when we got there. He had, after all, signed the lease (no, he replies, he never saw it). I tried to explain that all our things would meet us there, however these were now abstracts that didn't really make sense to him. He just wanted to know where I was taking him, but couldn't quite understand where that place was. I should mention that he lived in the Seattle area for a number of years in Bellevue, Marysville, and on Mercer Island. He had also driven that road between Bellevue and Plains on many, many occasions. Nothing sparked a memory.

Moses Lake was really peaceful. We had a huge room, a nearby reasonably priced restaurant and a view of the lake. I actually managed to accomplish quite a bit of work and he seemed relatively happy. Even then I was still trying to convey the concept of our things meeting us in Seattle. He just could not quite imagine the truck we saw in Calgary meeting us in Seattle and giving us all our things back. I guess the poor man thought that all his things had been taken from him and that his choice of destination was completely out of his control. Well, in truth, that was partly correct.

The last morning on the road, a Saturday, we made the short hop to Bellevue. We checked into our room and I drove us to the house to look around. The landlord was still working on the place and it seemed in total disarray. Knowing the truck wasn't due until Monday at the earliest, I felt like we might work it out, although I was a bit dubious. After all, I had paid for access effective the first and here it was the tenth. There was, however, nothing to worry about. In fact, we had found one of the most wonderful landlords we had ever had. He helped us sort out some personal things so that I could continue to work while I waited for my own internet connection to be established the next day. My husband could not understand that the house was ours, that the man would eventually be gone and that this was where our things would be delivered just any day.

We had to live in the hotel room for three days waiting for the truck. Truthfully, I was nearly at the end of my rope. It is never easy living in a motel. It was also difficult to work from a house that wasn't really ours yet. And, there was no way to make these issues clear to my husband. We did have an interesting moment the night before we expected things to arrive. I had explained to him that we would move into the house to stay the next day. He decided we needed to load as much as we could. At first I was a bit slow and thought he wanted to go right then, but no, he was only trying to make it easier for the morning. Moments of lucidity...

It was during our stay in that over-crowded, dark hotel room in Bellevue that, after crawling in bed for the night, he said: "I don't know what I would do without you. I just realized how much I need you." I don't know if everyone gets these precious moments in the midst of chaos, but I have learned to grasp them and cherish them and remember them during the moments that spike the stress meter.

When our long awaited possessions did arrive, he couldn't understand why things were just left here and there. It was a total mess, what were those people thinking? The first day or so he was so worried about having a place to work he started to set up the bedroom next to my office as a place for himself. It appeared that until I started to unpack the 300 or so boxes we had and he could see his office emerging, he would not be "settled."

Again, once the process was started he could be left on his own with several boxes of books and he would quietly work away. I noticed the organization was a bit different. For instance, color and size seemed more important in groupings than subject. I could not get him to understand that files went in file cabinets and books went on bookshelves. I finally ended up typing up one of my now famous sheets so if "that woman" told him any differently he had something to show her. Also, we were back at the game of "no, that's my book and it belongs on my shelves (even if it is a cookbook or talks about needlepoint or pottery)." My poor exercise bike got moved from room to room, upstairs and downstairs, driving me to near distraction and often causing the risk of bodily damage (ours, not the bike's). And, then, at last I managed to get it back in the room I wanted it. It seems happy there, now. I hope.

Finding a New "Normal"

There were a number of people who could not understand why I would drag a library consisting of well over 2,000 books and probably 100 boxes of files 750 miles across international borders. Well, it was because as long as he has his "stuff" and can "work," he is relatively stable and I can avoid making that most devastating of decisions to place him under longer term care. That decision also carries a cost for which I can no longer get insurance. It is my firm belief that for him, that type of care would be a death sentence; a place that would make him give up trying. Even in his current state of mind he still wants to read, he still asks questions and he still wants to tell other people what he is thinking. I believe the phrase for that return on investment is *"priceless."*

This may not be the case for everyone and the choice to seek outside help or to place a loved one under professional care can only be made by the person responsible for the ailing individual. No one can make that choice for you and you shouldn't let them. Although I have to admit, I was an active force in getting my father into long term care before my mother's health completely deteriorated. I think it boils down to whether or not the two of you still have and share a quality of life. Can you care for the medical issues (this was increasingly difficult for my mother)? How will you handle it if you come home to find he (or she) did not take a medication and you have a medical emergency on your hands? Can you sleep at night (something my mother was losing because my father would constantly call on her during the night)? My father also would refuse my mother's help for basic hygiene and had difficulty controlling his bowels; making the issue all that more difficult. So, do the inner smiles outpace the inner tears? Are you still able to learn about yourself and your loved one? Is your own physical and mental health still stable?

It's not just a character building exercise, there really is much to be said about seeing ourselves in a different way and stretching ourselves to accomplish things we never really thought of trying; like providing the richest end-of-life experience possible for the people nearest to us. That's when we learn what it is in life that matters to each of us most, and, believe me; it *is* priceless. Never, never allow yourself to feel guilty for the choice you make. Only you know your strengths and weaknesses and only you know what you are able to sacrifice. Sometimes seeking professional help *is* how you can best provide that "quality of life" for your loved one. The choice is yours and yours alone, make it and move on. Really. Listen to those that love you, but feel comfortable with the path you choose. And when it's time to try something different, then do so. My mother did.

We seem settled again. More or less. In the following pages I describe some of the more specific tools and insights I have developed. They include a bit more of the day to day issues that one deals with when living with a loved one afflicted with dementia. Through it all I have tried to stick to a few fundamental rules.

1. If you don't have a sense of humor you had better find one and quickly. You really need the ability to see the humor in the little dance your daily life becomes. Learn to laugh at yourself, as well.
2. "Remember" is no longer in the dictionary; neither is "explaining," "don't you see" or anything related to "logic."
3. Do everything in your power to defuse a situation. If you get agitated, your loved one will get agitated and any hope of a conversation or resolution will go right out the window. You will spend hours getting back to the status quo, and it is not worth the agitation and wasted emotion. That person cannot help it; don't act as if they can. There are times when I notice that a bit of grumpiness on my part helps deliver a message. However, be very careful that things don't escalate into an argument.
4. The question of whether or not to be honest with your loved one is discussed in depth in literature, both professional and private as it relates to many forms of dementia. Some say you must always be honest, although that will often cause arguments and alienation. Some say don't worry about it, they forget everything

anyway. My goal has been to try to strike a balance. How important is the question? Does the subject tend to upset the person, or is it something that for some reason seems important enough to them that they really want the answer? This one is a day to day, subject to subject question. I do not lie to my husband if I can possibly avoid it. I also will not sacrifice his peace of mind to meet some personal standard of inner integrity. I will explain more later.

Don't try to force yourself into a mold written by someone else, no matter how educated or experienced that person is. Each and every person with dementia is different. The professional help available is invaluable, but it must be applied with care and with an awareness of your specific situation, and your own inner convictions.

I also truly believe it is important that you don't try to fit yourself and your loved one into someone else's box. Each and every support resource has its own goals, qualifications and limitations. It is not your job to change their agenda; it is your job to find the organization or individual that fits in your box and within your limitations as best as can be accomplished.

Here, then are the lessons I have learned along the way. Some I must keep reminding myself of on a daily basis. Perhaps they will help others in their journey through never-never land. Keep in mind that many of these little insights overlap and cross over. There really isn't a chronological order so forgive me if it appears as though I am wandering. As you will see, each "facet" of this experience lights up another corner of our experience.

Show & Tell &Tolkien Languages

Considering my husband, at his best, could speak and/or write in five ancient and five modern languages, it was a bit of a surprise to me when he started to "lose his nouns." At first it was a game for us. I would refuse to buy, find, or address something until he found the word. Amazingly, he could often give me two or three full dictionary-style definitions, but that elusive noun just would not come to his lips until sometime later. This started before we even left for Canada. I think it worried him even then since he would tell me that he contacted a doctor that he knew that specialized in the field of memory retention and that he had been tested. Everything seemed fine. I wonder now if that call and test were ever really made.

At some point I realized that our "game" was not going to work anymore. Most markedly after his fall that January. To keep peace and to function on a day to day basis I learned to play Show and Tell. So, when I was making a shopping list and he was trying to tell me what we were running out of: Show me. When we were in the store and he was trying desperately to describe something to me he needed: Show me; point to it when we go by. When he wanted something moved, or needed something fixed: Show me. Sometimes that became rather difficult. So, we switched to a game of "what does it do?" "Tell me what you would use it for." "Where would I keep it?" Even today we function using some modified version of charades. The point is you can't always communicate in the manner to which you have become accustomed.

There were other language difficulties. During the years before the real plunge, while we would sit and talk about ideas, people, and/or places, my husband would tend to leave out the subject of his sentence. We had been together so long that I could often fill in the blank; sometimes without thinking about it. At some point I grew concerned that I was missing the point completely or making assumptions that I should not so I tried to get him to "name the subject (of the sentence)." Again, long, nicely composed descriptions, no word, name or other noun. I also realized in later months that some of our arguments came from my need to fill in that blank; and his frustration with not being able to fill it. I wonder now; how often was it so important that I *know*? Or was it simply my defense mechanism refusing to see what was right before my eyes?

Our communication difficulties increased dramatically after that trip to Vancouver Island. Suddenly, my husband found his nouns, but they were not in any dictionary I was familiar with. Having only studied French and Latin I cannot determine if these words are combinations of various nouns and verbs from some other place or time or some other jumble of sounds in his mind. I do know that he can look at me and express a thought in clear, articulated sounds that all make sense, except for that pesky noun. What is scary is that sometimes I do understand what he is trying to say. At least whatever my response is at the time seems to be satisfactory. He used to tease me with Hawaiian words and phrases and at first I thought that was the source. Now, I am no longer sure where these strange vocalizations come from: maybe they are from a land of Tolkien's imagination.

Since I am such an avid reader, I have experienced a number of times when I know perfectly well what a word is and how it sounds; but what comes out of my mouth isn't quite what I hear in my head. It takes a certain amount of practice to get what we hear in our heads to agree with what we vocalize. Perhaps this is a bit of what is happening to him. His brain is forgetting how to make the sounds he hears perfectly well within his own head. I say this because he is so certain of himself while he is talking; it is much different from when he couldn't find the word. So, has he simply stopped trying to match sound with thought, or is the thought now completely destroyed and he fills in the blanks as best he can?

There are some sounds that seem to attract him, much like a child. Bam Bam from the Flintstones comes to mind. When I crack an egg, close a door, bang a pot or pan; I often hear "bang, bang" behind me. He will, at times, try to repeat other sounds he hears. There are certain decibels that reach his ears loud and clear with or without his hearing aids. He does, for instance, hear the bearing that is going out in our car even though at this point it is merely that distant moan that rises and falls with the speed of the car. I think what I have found is that the level of communication within the brain cannot always be determined by the communication level with the outside world. It just isn't always useful to judge the mental capacity of a person based solely on their ability to express his or hers inner thoughts.

We watched a movie recently, *Hitch*. In the narration the main character explains that some 90% or more of all human communication is non-verbal. Thank goodness. If I have learned anything from this part of our relationship it is that communication is still vital. It may not take place in the ways that we were accustomed to; it may be a guessing game of sorts from time to time. It is, however, both possible and necessary. As long as you develop the attitude to seek those avenues and accomplish the end goal with the least amount of emotional turmoil for yourself and your loved one.

So, for your own peace of mind you need to find avenues of communication that work. There is an idea that is necessary to communicate somewhere in your loved one's head. Try to find a non-confrontational way of getting that idea communicated and acted on. Try also to avoid humiliating or degrading the person. As far as they are concerned everything they say is perfectly understandable; you are the one with the problem. After all, as he says from time to time, it may really be a Japanese word...

Prodigal Pronouns

One of the dramatic changes that occurred when we returned from the Island was the use of pronouns. To this day I get in trouble with this issue. There can never be a "we," and "he" and "she" need to leave the house. There is only "you" and "me." Every other pronoun leads to all kinds of issues about who was where when, who is taking me/us where, how many people are expected (none) and several other interpretive scenarios. There are times when I end up quite confused myself.

This may have something to do with the inability to understand abstracts, to put names to things that are not physically present. It might also come from his long years of literal translations in the world of mathematics and physics. "We" can mean all sorts of things and it does not have to be limited to those present and accounted for. Since he thinks of me as a whole team of people running around and taking care of him, "we" can be and sometimes is me. When you speak with someone suffering with dementia, clearly identify the parties involved without "talking down." You and I will go to dinner; you and I will go to the doctor. No, I don't know where "she" (or he) is, so you and I will go to the store.

Time is an Essence

Although this concept is finally making its way into my thick head it is probably the one issue I still have a major problem with. An individual with dementia cannot comprehend abstracts; which means there is no time. There is no yesterday, tomorrow can be a really tough problem, and if they have an issue right now, there is nothing on this earth that can possibly be more important. Think two-year old.

Since I have managed, for the most part, to work from home up to now, I tend to be rather focused during the hours I am being paid. I also try to work on small accounts during weekends and evenings. Most of the time I can handle the several little things that come up in the course of caring for him during day and keep on going. Sometimes, however, it is just not possible. It is so much easier to just drop everything, take care of the issue (if that is actually possible) and then go back to whatever was going on in relative peace. Why I have such an issue learning that simple process I'm really not sure.

Here are a few examples. A few weeks after we were settled into our new home my husband decided he needed to get into a fire safe file cabinet that he had not been in for probably two years. There is no telling where the key may have gone. This is not a simple file cabinet. It is a fire safe that requires a licensed locksmith to come to the house and give the manufacturer his license number so that he can receive drilling instructions and break into the safe; hopefully without damaging the $150-200 lock. Can we wait two days so I can check a few more boxes for the keys? No! Can we wait until later in the day after I am done working so I can make some phone calls and get prices? No! It must be now, right now, and I (my husband) am not going to pay for it! It's not my fault! (I see).

This particular little adventure was a bit costly. There were others, and it always ends up in a long drawn out conversation of what is or is not happening or when "she" or "we" or "he" are going to get things done. Big sigh, move on. It really is best to stop for a few minutes and think about the cost of escalating the situation. The wear and tear on your emotions (and his/hers) is really not worth whatever little bit of something you manage to finish (or mess up) while trying to put off the inevitable. In our case there is sometimes a long conversation on why it is not necessary for him to find someplace else to live. We can and will work this particular issue out and continue to live together. Is this really the kind of conversation to which you need to devote some portion of your day? Probably not. Learn to allocate time to useful pursuits that move things along in a more serene fashion.

This same concept applies to expressing future plans. It is highly recommended that you don't start the morning with, "You and I are going to the store this afternoon." Not good. It will be afternoon all day. You always need to give the person enough time to prepare, dress, shave, whatever, but not so much that the process of going takes up the whole day. There are times when it is important to express later time commitments; however, try to find a balance between giving notice and devoting all of the time before the appointment to explaining why the two of you haven't left yet. Or, learn to repeat the time you leave many, many times without getting upset or distressed. Sometimes my husband will get confused and decide we were not going after all. If it is a short trip I may go myself, or I might reschedule. Time in a bottle; it changes shape with each day and experience.

I have also worked out a few ways to deal with the "later" and "tomorrow" thing. If I discover a date or appointment has become rather important to him I will make sure that he sees it on the calendar. Then we mark each day off as it goes by. This is a way of "counting" to a point in the future when he will see the doctor, when we are going somewhere specific, when the truck is coming to take all our things away.

While we were still in Canada and I was working downtown half a day I developed a weekly calendar that I hung on the wall in the kitchen. That way he knew when I was leaving, when I would call, when I was coming home, and how long I was expected to work once I was home. By the way, I used my proper name throughout, no "she," "her," or "me." This gave us consistency, a point of reference for him and a place I could point to if he lost track of things. Of course, every now and then "someone" would make him move that schedule. When I catch up with "her," "she" will definitely get a piece of my mind! Wait, "she" already has it...

Practicing the approach of "time in a bottle" is beginning to work through my system. Not so long ago he came to me near the lunch hour and announced we had to leave right that minute. The battery in his watch had been acting up for about a day and I had promised to take him to the store that afternoon to get it fixed. Suddenly that wasn't good enough. It had to be now; right now. After deciding this was one of those times when surrender was the better part of valor I shut down my computer and off we went. I think, like say a five-year-old, something in his mind said, "Oops, I think I went too far, and she is *really* not happy." He suggested that if it was going to take a while I could leave him there and come back later (yeah, right). He apologized a number of times and offered to help with the garbage bins when we returned. During the afternoon he was very helpful and was obviously trying to make up for what he gathered was not a good move. I have to admit that I was a bit smug. Somehow I had communicated that this was not the best way to handle things. Whether that "lesson" will carry forward into any future activity or not; well I'm not holding my breath. The good thing is that when we did get back home I could jump in and complete the item I was working on fairly quickly and my own mental state was: "Hey, it really does work!"

There is another issue that I believe fits into the concept of "time as an essence." There is a condition called "sundowners," or "sundown syndrome" that occurs when an elderly person becomes depressed, agitated or confused during the nighttime hours. After observing my husband, I firmly believe that this condition has something to do with the failure to grasp time. My husband used to get up in the middle of the night, put on a robe and disappear into his office to write. I can understand that. I have been known to keep a notebook by my bed during intense negotiations because a resolution to a particular issue would often come to me in a semi-sleep mode that I would lose if I didn't write it down. "Sundowning" does not appear to be related to this sort of behavior.

What happens now is that my husband may spring out of bed at 1:30 in the morning fully convinced that the night is over. He prefers to go to bed around 7:00 which means, really, that he probably has had enough sleep: not so with me since I probably didn't go to bed until 9:00 or 10:00. I find that the more I try to convince him that it is the middle of the night, the less cooperation I get. Even if I insist that I need more sleep, well, he'll spend an hour telling me how much I need it which doesn't really produce the intended result.

I have to admit that the few nights we have had to deal with this I was worried. A person needs sleep. Sleepy people do not make good accountants or financial analysts. Such an issue is part of the reason I was able to convince my mother that it was time to move my father into care. There is, however, a major difference between the two cases. My father demanded that my mother pop up and get this, fix that or take care of something else. I have found that my husband will let me stay in bed and sleep. We did have to come to an agreement.

The morning that worried me the most, he got up, turned on the lights, and decided he needed his shower. That entails that I get up. Once I started his shower I tried napping on the couch; without success. After he realized his error and decided we should go back to bed (about an hour or so later) we worked out a deal. If he felt it was necessary to get up, fine. However, don't turn on the lights and demand showers. Lately I have been able to sleep through the middle of the night excursions. At least for now.

I admit this is not hard for me because I have always been a light sleeper. Waking just enough to check on things and falling back into dream mode is a habit honed over decades. This is not a one size fits all and I have no idea if our "deal" will stick. As I keep pointing out in this story, it is a dance that must take into consideration the changing landscape of your lives.

Stealing Mail

For the first several weeks after our return from the Island my husband seemed to be almost desperate to separate me from "her." If we stopped to pick up the mail he would get his but he saw no reason for me to have or even look at "hers." This could pose a problem. Most of our personal business was handled on-line, but there were papers and bills I needed to have. So, the solution was to steal the mail. This is not difficult since few houses receive their mail at the front door any more, and if it is an issue I suggest you open a box at a local store or post office. Try to communicate via email as much as you can. Yes, it costs a bit for a box; however, what is the cost of missing a notice on insurance, losing a title or registration, or some letter from social security or some other agency (like Canadian immigration)? My husband did, finally, get comfortable with my going through the mail and he seems comfortable now that I process mail in "her" name. I do try to pick things I can give him such as magazines, notices addressed to him I am already aware of, anything that indicates he is still part of the process.

For the most part, I learned to find a work-around so that we could function, I would be aware of important developments, and I didn't fight him or impact his dignity. Extra work? Not really. Cleaning up the emotional blow back after a struggle of this sort is far more time consuming than just finding a different perspective.

The Magic Desk & Other Disappearing Acts

Another hill that was difficult for me personally was when things started to move. Books I had carefully collected over a number of years were suddenly his. So much his that he stamped his name on them (shudder) and would move them to his library and out of my office. Since our interests were so similar in a number of areas, it was sometimes understandable. I don't recall, however, that he ever had an interest in needlepoint or pottery making.

I have always been a private person, and the few things that have traveled life with me are precious to me. Some of these books were important to me for research purposes, some of them were business texts I needed for work. Whatever the subject I had to work through my mind that they really were not going anywhere; at least not far. And although I do shudder when someone marks a book (too many years working in the book trade and seeing the value decline because of a mark or missing jacket) I was able to trade that "ownership" for my husband's peace of mind. Most of the time. The only thing I worried about was that he would decide to throw something away because *he* didn't want it any more. It does pay to keep an eye on the trash.

The other area I am very protective of is my desk. It is, after all, an office and often has information that is important to my clients and should not be "shared." So, when something goes missing I get a bit uptight. Such a thing happened soon after our return from the Island. A stack of papers that had been on the corner of my desk for months (mostly to do with us, but not entirely) suddenly disappeared. "Where did the papers go, dear?" "What papers?"

Not remembering entirely what was in that stack I went into overdrive and checked other spots on my desk. I learned where he would poke and what he would not look at and where to keep things put away. I did finally find the papers several weeks later in a briefcase in our bedroom. What you need to understand is that at that point he thought his "wife" was not coming back. That meant that anything on "her" desk was fair game. Some of it had his name on it and he felt the need to protect that information. These were his things: my panic was meaningless to him.

I highly recommend that you look at your things, the pieces that make up your lives, and if there is anything that you do not want broken, lost, moved, marked or changed in anyway, tuck them away somewhere for future caring. This is a delicate process because, first of all, you have these things because you enjoy them and, secondly, your loved one might wonder where your mind has gone if you start squirreling away all your precious memories. They may feel frustrated because they can no longer locate important documents. It is a dance; as is every aspect of life with a failing mind. When things are peaceful and you can walk through the choices you have, decide what is worth the risks and what is not. Then when the emotional moment comes you are better prepared to deal with the consequences: even watching precious, out of print books being stamped with someone's name or losing a dust jacket.

Fixing the Coffee Pot

My husband, for years, has fixed the coffee while I showered and got ready for work. We would eat breakfast together and I would drive off for another day in the "Core." Sometime after our return from the island, I noticed that the amount of coffee grounds he used increased dramatically and that there was often water or coffee running off the counter. And yet, and he would still be worrying over the coffee pot. I thought he had forgotten how to make coffee. Well, yes and no. What was happening was that the coffee pot was giving up and no matter how much water (or coffee) he put in, the carafe would not fill. He was fixing the coffee pot. I bought a new one.

After that we both made coffee. It was another case, at first, of not solving the problem because I didn't know the question. I kept insisting he was putting too much coffee in. I wasn't taking the time to figure out that he was trying to make more coffee because the coffee pot wasn't making enough. Again, communication is not easy, but when something is frustrating your beloved, try to see what end result they are seeking. For instance, he doesn't turn off a light when he doesn't understand the switch (like the in-line wheels), he just unplugs it. It took him six weeks to learn how to turn off the dimmer switch in our new dining room. But guess what, he did learn.

Another concept that left his mind is why coffee pots automatically shut off. He thought ours was broken because it would not keep his coffee hot all day. So he would turn it back on and it would steam away without water and finally wear out the mechanism. Something else that had slipped by me is that somewhere along the line the function and use of the microwave had drifted out of his mind. I did try writing notes, (Press 115 Start to warm a cup of coffee), but that only worked for a while. I have elected to purchase cheaper coffee pots: then it doesn't hurt the pocket so much when the poor things give up in a cloud of steam. I also try to catch him when he starts looking for that cup of coffee and warm it up for him. Whereupon he asks if he can watch so that he can learn how to do it. Why not? He just might.

Another odd reaction to modern day coffee pots is his insistence that the digital read out is a temperature, not a time indicator. I have tried to explain the function of a clock in a coffee pot, but he is certain I have lost my marbles. He assumes that as the numbers go up, the coffee will be warmer, or more "ready." Thus, I continue to warm his coffee whenever I notice he is looking for another cup.

It also became necessary for me to try to take out the garbage. He actually still considers that his job, but the difference between recycle and trash is beyond him. His office wastebasket will often get emptied into the bin of the moment without a bag. At one point he told me that the things that went in the blue bin were for people who needed those things and someone had stolen them from our front yard.

Washers and dryers and dishwashers have now become mysteries as well. He still, though, wants to learn. Consequently, he asks me to show him how to do this or that. Keep in mind it does not matter if the person will actually "learn" how to complete the task. The point is they asked. They are still interested, and whether your lesson sticks or not, curiosity is a spark of life you will learn to treasure. Teach, every day if you must, showing that kind of interest and support can do wonders. And, no, don't respond by saying, "I've already shown you how to do that a thousand times!" Unless, of course, you enjoy starting arguments and confrontations!

Buying Clothes & Other Closet Adventures

My husband was not really a clotheshorse in earlier years, but he did like to dress well. He had excellent taste in colors and combinations and would always appreciate it when I found something just right for him. During our transitional period a number of things began to happen.

First of all the collars on his shirts became too tight. My husband is a very thin person and has continued to lose weight. His neck, however, has thickened. For some reason he feels he must have a shirt or sweater or pull-over right around his neck. This required moving buttons, buying new shirts or tops and finding buttons that his increasingly arthritic fingers could manipulate. A man that never used to swear, even with euphemisms, suddenly became quite colorful when it came to getting clothes on and off.

As mentioned, he used to be delighted when I found something I thought was in his color range. He also took very good care of his clothes, undoing buttons before washing, hanging and folding things in a certain way, asking for help when one thing or another needed a bit of repair. I started to notice changes not too long before we left for the Island.

First of all, it seemed important to him to keep his coats in the bedroom closet rather than in the coat closet by the garage. I'm not sure if this was a territorial thing or if he just wanted things where he would see them and remember where they were. During the packing for our move he was very distraught because the movers had put the mattress in front of the closet and he could not get to the 3 or 4 things that were still there. After finally understanding what the issue was, I had to climb over the mattress and hand him the hangers with those few items. Bearing them proudly before him he announced to the movers that they were his and it was okay for him to have them. A heart-stopping moment for me.

After our return from the Island, I also noticed a bit of confusion about what was what. He would get dressed in one of his light-weight jackets with no shirt. The jacket would be tucked into his jeans and zippered to the top. We had purchased a fuzz-lined hoody for warmth on cooler days, this suddenly became a shirt. He would often wear multiple layers and sometimes come to bed fully dressed. The difference between pajamas and day clothes appeared to be somewhat lost at times.

He did have one pair of pajamas that he liked. Keeping in mind that throughout our marriage pajamas had not been a priority, this pair suddenly became a nightly ritual. Since he liked clean pajamas, I tried to find some alternatives. He also had a second set that was several years old. No new pajamas seemed to work for more than a night or two. I think, in retrospect, at least one problem was that the patterns and colors were confusing. They looked too much like other things he wore. At first it seemed that he didn't want to make a mistake and wear the wrong thing, so he stayed with the pair that was different from everything else. He would only wear the alternatives when his favorite pair was just not available and sometimes not at all. We now make sure that his favorite ones are washed every other day.

As noted above, he was always a very organized person when it came to his clothing (as opposed to, say, his files). After our arrival back in Seattle I sorted out the boxes that had his clothes in them. He only unpacked about half of them. He put some shirts in drawers, rumbled his tee shirts and underwear into drawers and kept only those things he could figure out on hangers. Now that I think about it, he usually did ask my advice regarding what he should wear to this or that office or to run some errand. Now it appeared that he wanted that advice more specifically. He can still dress himself, he just needs a little guidance from time to time regarding what he should actually wear.

When this becomes a problem, try suggesting changes, rather than blurting out something like, "Whatever possessed you to dress like that?" Something like, "You may be more comfortable in that," or "For this visit you may want to wear this," gets things moving much faster and in the right direction. Don't make the issue confrontational. At least in my case that always resulted in a "equal and opposing force" moment.

Sometimes when I would purchase new clothes for him, I couldn't get him to wear them. One way I solved this problem was to simply mix things in. We had purchased a new pair of jeans because he was losing so much weight a lot of things were hanging on him. They fit well, but he seemed hesitant to wear them. So, I washed them and mixed them in with other pairs in his closet. He almost caught me. When he first took them out of the closet he said that he didn't remember having this pair. Then he decided his son had borrowed them and must have sent them back. Whatever works, my dear, whatever works. But how in the world did he remember, out of two dozen pairs of jeans, that particular pair was new? The wonders of the human mind... Now he has decided all these clothes were left for him, not his to begin with.

Recently, I discovered that I was, in part, again attempting to solve the wrong problem. One evening as he got prepared for bed, he didn't want his favorite pajamas because they should be washed (every other day). We started a conversation about what was available for him to wear to bed and it was rather enlightening. One, he did not like ties on the pants, he preferred snaps, well actually he preferred elastic waistbands. Two, the top should come up closer to his neck when it buttoned. We had a conversation about telling me these things while we were shopping. He said he didn't want to be a bother and I tried to explain that it was preferable to be a bother rather than spend money on things a person didn't want. Grab the moments of lucidity when they come, you will treasure each one more than you can imagine.

Another problem that developed in our "closet adventures" is where certain things were kept. No matter how often he was shown, he could not remember where to find toilet paper, cotton balls, rubbing alcohol, facial tissue... Believe me, it's far easier if you just stop and show, point or retrieve it yourself. Sometimes pointing doesn't work too well either. Saying, "That's in the hall closet," "look under the sink" (where it's always been) or any other directional information usually does not result in the item being found. You save a lot of time and effort if you just say, "Oh, that's right over here. Let me help you find it," and go get it. If you are patient, there are occasions when directions work. Recently, while working in our yard, I decided to give it a try and send him into the house for a cap to keep the hair out of my eyes as I worked. Well, he got the right closet but the first choice I was offered was one of my jackets vs. one of his. When I explained, and pantomimed something for my head, he returned with a choice of caps. It's a matter of timing (good and comfortable moods) and approach; "Yes, dear you could help. I need a cap."

Personal Hygiene & Other Cleaning Guides

This subject differs so much from person to person that there can only be some general pieces of advice and a sharing of my own experience. My husband has always been very meticulous about cleanliness. One should wash one's hands after handling garbage (still does), one should bath daily (still does), one should make sure that clothes are clean and tidy (mostly still does). It is now necessary for me to wash the clothes although he had done it for several years. It is also now necessary for me to set up his shower water. We have gone from one knob to three and he can't quite get the water temperature where he wants it. I have learned things such as "too heavy" means "too hot." There was one major problem as we entered this stage in his live and that was with his teeth.

His teeth were never really in great shape, but as he aged and as his cardiovascular system developed problems, the need for dental health became more than a commercial for a smile. Even though I walked through several procedures a number of times, and even though he would watch me every morning through my routine, after his decline on the Island the whole process seemed to mystify him. He understood the value of dental health. He did have medical training. But somehow he couldn't translate that into action. When he was going through the pre-surgery interview for a hernia repair in 2011 the anesthesiologist almost declined the surgery because of his dental health. They were going to use a mesh which is, after all, a foreign body which can and does collect unwanted bacteria. The doctor told me that if he was going in for a joint replacement he would have been denied flat out.

With that in mind we picked up a Waterpic to see if he could get more focused on his teeth. I had to help him every time he used it (while trying not to shower the whole bathroom) and eventually he just refused. When I asked him if he was brushing his teeth the answer was "of course." I wonder where that constant supply of toothpaste came from and how it was that he could use the brush that was still in the package.

My dentist refused to work on his mouth at all, both because of his history of seizures and because of his cardiovascular health. We did visit a denture clinic for advice, but the cost of replacing even one plate was beyond our budget.

These sorts of decisions are really tough. Do you really need a daily fight to get something done? He was worried because when he brushed his teeth they bled. I tried to explain that yes, they would. They were diseased and needed more cleaning. When we moved back to Seattle, I made sure his insurance included dental. Maybe now a doctor can work on his teeth and salvage something if only to protect his heart.

There is no specific advice one can provide on such an issue. It is a family affair. The best advice I can offer is that for the things that you can handle, haircuts, nail trimming, bathing, whatever, keep after it in a gentle but firm manner. If it has to do with something that will cause constant contention or that you do not have the skill to handle, look for a day nurse or senior service that can perform the procedure for you. Sometimes the cost can be a bit high. I know when I checked on having a nurse do his toe nails (he does have some issues with his feet) it was something like $72.00 for a minimum of one hour. For now I think I can work on his nails.

Another man-thing is shaving. For our entire relationship my husband has shaved every morning and sometimes in the evening if we were going somewhere. At some point that I can't quite pin down, shaving became a once-every-day-or-so thing. Purchasing a razor also became an issue because I was never sure if he wasn't using it correctly or if there really was a problem. Electric razors are not particularly cheap. Perhaps some of the problem is that he used to be very meticulous about cleaning his razor every single day. It could be that without this type of maintenance, things just didn't function as they should. In any event, it wasn't difficult to get him to shave if we were going somewhere and if he was given sufficient notice. I chose not to make an issue out of it. It is rather odd that for a month or so he chose to carry the razor around with him when he "went to work" in the morning, along with the case for his glasses and his "ears."

Recently, however, this situation became much clearer and I discovered another instance of solving the wrong problem. It all came to a head late one afternoon when he brought the razor to me because it wasn't working and he didn't know how to clean it, and the charge had run down. Who knows where the manual was. We managed to get it cleaned and charged but then he wanted to go to the doctor, not next week: tomorrow. All because of some vague pain or something on his neck. There is some sense in this as he did suffer from rashes in the past when things were not maintained correctly; however I had some difficulty explaining that the doctor could not fix the razor. It is also the case that when shaving is not a regular thing razor rash or other skin irrigations can be very uncomfortable, especially under tight collars, which is probably why he thought that a doctor might be needed to solve the issue.

Thank goodness for the internet. I was able to locate and print a manual for his razor. Still not quite enough. So, with a bit more patience and persistent questioning, I discovered that what was really wrong is that he had forgotten how to shave. Not, necessarily how to run the razor back and forth across his face, but all the things before and after that make shaving a successful enterprise. So, off to the internet again and I found step by step instructions on how a fellow should shave with an electric shaver. After getting a bit more education I could explain that I did understand the issue and could fix it. I promised to take him the very next day (after work) to find the correct things to help him accomplish his goal. This time he waited. I also used the situation to suggest that maybe he should shave every day. He has quite oily skin and it is clear how problems could arise rather quickly. Another lesson in learning to "hear" whether or not it is actually being "said." Even if it takes coaching on a regular basis this was something that was important enough to make sure that he followed through on a regular routine.

That routine quickly morphed into my own barber shop. At some point I realized that he firmly believed that he had not been plagued with all that prickly stuff when he lived "up there." Within a few weeks I found that it was easier if I performed the ritual of shaving for him. Honestly, I actually enjoy it. It provides meaningful physical contact and a chance to reinforce our bond.

I do not, at this point, have to bathe him. This was necessary while the fracture he had suffered in Plains was healing. We managed pretty well with a shower seat and a hand held shower head. I would suppose that bathing your beloved is much easier if you are a spouse than it might be if, say, you are a caregiver for your parent. Again, this is a personal choice and if you are not comfortable for any reason, get professional help. You cannot let someone's health deteriorate because you are squeamish about bubbles and bottoms and other parts.

Good health is, of course, more than personal hygiene. I can remember some years ago when he was surprised I was cleaning the bathrooms. For some reason he thought the landlord was supposed to do that. Boy, don't I wish! He also had allergies that made it important for me to have him somewhere else when I dusted and vacuumed (although in later years even with warning he would simply follow me around the house). Recently, for some reason, having him in some other part of the house while I vacuumed became a problem. As is my habit, I let him know that I was going to clean house and would be running the vacuum. All of a sudden he needed to walk around the block or move somewhere else. After much conversation I convinced him to stay in the house (and continue to live with me) until I was ready to vacuum and then he could walk around in our yard. Next time I will know better and won't mention vacuums and such until the last minute. Or, wait until his new companion takes him off for a hour or so.

He still helps me with the dishes, though not as much, and we both take out the trash. It is important, I think, that you not make the person feel useless, pushing them away or saying you don't need help. No matter how trivial, there should be something he or she can do to help, and it makes a huge difference in his or her self esteem. That translates into easier handling of other problems.

Medical Issues & Playing Nurse

This is one of those areas that can be a deciding moment for any care giver when it comes to choosing professional help or full time care. My husband is basically healthy. He does have a stent; however stress tests in the last several years have indicated that his cardiovascular health is stable. As mentioned above, he does have a controlled seizure disorder. This means that he has a combination of medications and over-the-counter things that he should take on a daily basis. Sometimes that works; sometimes it gets hairy. I have, from time to time, ordered new prescriptions with a different doctor's name because he was upset with the doctor. For instance, the neurologist that indicated he had a serious memory issue and should be assessed by the Cognitive Assessment Center. Anything with that doctor's name on it was a losing battle, so I had the prescription reissued by our primary care physician.

I also try to make things as habitual as I can. We both take our medications during breakfast and dinner and he gets a glass of water to help with some of the larger pills. He does, from time to time, put up an argument. The only prescription that worries me during these momentary battles is the anti-convulsant. The choice I had to make was whether or not I should make this a daily fight or if I should deal with the issue as best I could and hope that he maintained enough in his system. Seizures are not normally life-threatening, unless something happens to the individual during the seizure, such as a fall, choking or smothering. I have been present during two of his seizures. The first frightened me immensely. The second I was well read up and prepared. It's a decision that each caregiver must make for him or herself. If it were some other life-supporting drug I would most likely be faced with seeking some kind of professional help. In the meantime, we work it out as best we can and he follows the protocol the majority of the time.

There was a time when he blamed some of his prescriptions for impacting his mental capacity. Did he know that something was happening and consequently looked for any cause external to himself that he could control? I will never know. I do know that I made a commitment to him that I would never try to pass something off on him that I knew he had concerns about. And, I won't. That is part of my inner ethics.

New and wonderful drugs are being developed to help stabilize people with various forms of dementia and memory loss. The use of these prescriptions is a choice on a case by case basis. The medical profession really doesn't know all of the side effects these things can or might produce, but they do know some of them. The possibility of putting my husband on a memory boosting drug was discussed with our doctor, our pharmacist, an RN with geriatric experience, and his son.

The problem with some of these drugs if that if the patient misses even one dose the chances of a seizure increase to a statically significant number. And such an event is certain to plunge the patient further into the illness. My husband already suffers from the risk of seizure and I sometimes have difficulty making sure he takes the required medications. It was a risk/benefit ratio that neither I nor my stepson was comfortable with. Thus, it is a path we have not pursued. That does not mean it may not be a wise course for another family, another patient, another situation.

Another area that became difficult with my husband is determining symptoms. Once communication starts to lose its edge, it becomes very difficult to determine what exactly is going on. While we were working on getting a hernia repair scheduled, it was difficult to determine what was hurting how much. The hernia itself was diagnosed early in 2011. We did get surgery scheduled soon after our return from our vacation. Although I was happy we were going to get it handled before he could no longer communicate pain and recovery precisely, it was a bit of a circus accomplishing the end goal.

This is one of those times when the calendar became a counting machine. I also had to keep a picture of the surgeon handy because he kept getting confused about who was going to do the surgery. He had told me he liked the surgeon so I tried to keep it straight for him. This was at the time I hadn't yet learned that he often confused other people (as well as me) and assumed I was talking about one person when it was someone else altogether different. At one point I was afraid I was going to have to fight for the surgery because there was some concern that he wasn't capable of consenting. Our primary care physician wrote a letter to the hospital explaining that when the hernia was diagnosed he and my husband had a conversation about the various procedures and the risks and in his opinion my husband was an informed patient. (Whew).

He actually did fairly well with the initial stages of things and I stayed by his bedside until they wheeled him off for surgery. I tried to get some exercise and walk a bit until they returned him to the intake room. They told me I would not be permitted in recovery. I said fine, even though I had a inkling things weren't going to work according to their plans. Soon after the tracking board indicated he was out of surgery I wandered back to the intake room where I was told to expect to see him. A nurse came looking for me. He was quite agitated and they wondered if I would mind coming to recovery to help him work through the process. No problem, as I mentioned, I had rather expected it. He insisted nothing had happened, nothing had been fixed, and he still hurt. "Yes, dear, I know. They poked a hole in your tummy and it will hurt for a bit."

Recovery at home went very well. We managed to deal with the dressing and I stayed with him a full 24 hours after surgery. It was still difficult to judge pain levels. He had never been one to complain much about pain. Due to an old back injury he was fairly accustomed to it, so when he told me he hurt I knew it really hurt. The problem is that with the drugs he was on we had to be careful with the painkillers prescribed.

Luckily, we had no problems working around the dressing or bathing in a manner that would protect the bandage.

There are some cases when a person with dementia has difficulty understanding why they are all bandaged up and may not be willing to let things be for the required period of time. Keep in mind, he had no clue from where he had acquired or why he had acquired those staples in his head in January. It is really important to judge how cooperative your loved one will be so that you can avoid any real disasters such as infection, a reopening of the incision or further damage to the repair. At this point I was very lucky and he was very cooperative.

The next event did cause me some difficulty. I had been scheduled for a colonoscopy for nearly nine months. It would not be wise to put it off or cancel. I had to figure out how to get me to the hospital and back and not leave the car in the garage. He might decide to come looking for me and become disturbed because he didn't know where I was or why I wasn't calling. We went over and over what was planned for two or three days before the test. Obviously, I had preparations to make which he was certain were no longer needed. According to him, I must be going to some uninformed doctor. I scheduled a taxi to take us and bring us back. It was within a week or two of our return from the Island and he was still not certain of who I was so it was a bit of a dance to have him come with me; he wasn't quite sure why I would want him there. I typed everything up and made sure he had at least two numbers to reach our friends should something go awry or should he have questions about what was going on. When we got up the next morning he was completely confused. He called our friend (thank goodness it wasn't too early) and she talked him through the whole process. We got dressed and, holding tightly to his paper, we hopped into the taxi and went off to the hospital.

When I had been in that hospital almost a year earlier, they had let him stay in the recovery room while I was having an upper GI. Evidently the rules had changed and they wanted him in the hall. I asked the desk if I could talk that over with someone and they indicated that the nurse would make the decision. When she showed up her decision was, no, we had to follow rules. So I retrieved his instruction sheet and went over everything on the paper one more time and emphasized that if he had any questions or wondered where I was he should call our friend. "Ah, ha," says the nurse. "I think it would be better if he stayed right here with me. I will keep an eye out for any problems and help him if he needs anything." Then, with a bit of a smile and a wink she asked me, "Will this young man be driving you home?" Suddenly all the tension went out of me and I started to laugh. "No," I told her, "I didn't think I could pull that off!"

It is important for any caregiver to keep in mind that you will not be healthy every day all day. Sometimes you get sick. Sometimes it is something you can deal with like a cold, but sometimes it can be something really awful. After the fall but before our vacation, we were at the hospital trying to get a diagnosis on his hernia. We were there for hours and somewhere along the line I picked up some incredibly ugly flu. I was so sick I couldn't manage to get off the couch the next day where I was trying to stay away from him as much as I could. He wouldn't let me rest because he thought we should be at the hospital. (Please no, I don't want to catch anything else)! I finally called our primary care physician so that he could talk my husband into calming down and to tell him what to look for if I needed help. Peace. No more questions. Sleep, and eventually wellness. Too bad the cell phone was destroyed when I bathed in it alcohol to keep my husband from catching anything!

If you should become ill, don't try to take care of everything, answer questions and support your loved one. You have to rest to get well. At times like these it may be a good idea to have a number or two to call. So far I have been able to manage, but I have to take into account that if I am feeling bad he will get very worried and try to do something to make me better which does not include leaving me alone to suffer.

Another thing that happens to all of us as we age and things start to break down is difficulty controlling our bladders. It is evident this is a problem for a large portion of the population or our pharmaceutical companies would not be pressing "fix it" drugs on us during our favorite shows at night. It is a given. Be prepared. Added to this particular problem in our case is that my husband does not usually care to use public restrooms. Sometimes there really is no choice and in some places he seems relatively comfortable with the prospect; such as in restaurants.

I have learned to plan shopping and errand outings in smaller chunks, say 3-4 hours at most. It also seems wise to guide by example and make a stop at the bathroom before we leave. I have also learned that when he says he needs to go home then that is what we must do: go home. Don't get upset or flustered about the issue. It is far better to hop in the car and go home than deal with the embarrassment that is sure to occur if someone you truly care about soils themselves in public. If an accident does happen, you know what? It can be cleaned up and it can be done with grace and tenderness.

This has never happened to us except in the car or at home. I believe that is the case because I pay attention to him and his reactions and do my best to protect his dignity. It is nothing more than what I know he would do for me if the situation was reversed. In fact, during the years I suffered from migraines and would become so terribly ill (at home and in the car) he did exactly that; cleaned up after me. Yes, there are commercial solutions to a weak bladder, however, would you enjoy a shopping trip with a "wet diaper?" If your loved one is willing to wear incontinence protection, that's wonderful. You should still keep their comfort level in mind if the protection becomes necessary.

Again it is important to try to sort out what your own reactions might be when the failings and mishaps of aging occur before it is an emotional tornado that only harms you and your loved one. If you need help, it really is OK; just don't blame your loved one for something they really cannot control.

And, sometimes, all the planning in the world cannot prepare you for reality.

One last thing to cover in the day to day workings of health care. My husband has always suffered from digestive track issues. From diverticulitis several years ago to a constant and persistent problem with diarrhea in the past year or so. What has become somewhat comical is trying to sort out when he has the problem and when the opposite is the problem. When you ask him the response is, "No, I don't believe so." Then a day or two later he is concerned that he has some terrible disease because he has trouble getting to the bathroom in time and wants to assure me I won't catch it. (I know dear. I don't think I'm susceptible).

He also cannot comprehend the instructions from the doctor that are provided to get samples and such. As you know, doctors love to collect body fluids and various forms of body wastes to test and poke and prod. I have finally worked out two methods to know whether or not we have one extreme or the other going on. One is to listen (yep) and one is to look (yep again). I do clean the bathrooms and I can determine if he is having a problem and medications need to be adjusted. Sorry, but chronic diarrhea can be a serious health issue and it needs to be controlled and monitored.

So, we are back at issue one: can you manage, or do you need help? If this is not something you can manage on your own, ask the doctor for alternatives. Find out if you can have a day nurse come in for medical testing purposes. At some point you do have to decide if you can manage these types of issues that are rather routine when you are dealing with an aging individual. Don't be embarrassed if you just can't manage: get help. But be prepared, there will be times when the not-so-pleasant things of life become rather common parts of your day to day tasks. If you've ever been a parent it will be something like a re-wind of those early years. Think *The Curious Case of Benjamin Button*.

Books & Magazines

Since it has already been mentioned that we have a private library of over 2,000 books, it is probably pretty clear that we have always been avid readers. One of the things that attracted me to this man is his never-ending wonder. His sense that the universe was a great big machine that needed to be taken apart and put back together again. There was never a subject that was too trivial for background research, even the purchase of a mobile home for his stays in Plains, Montana. Consequently, our marriage was, at least in part, a merger of a rather large pile of information on every subject found on the Dewey Decimal System. And, of course, neither one of us stopped buying books or magazines.

It is a habit that approaches other people's need for tobacco. For instance, when we were driving around Calgary one summer to find a floor plan we could consider our dream house a friend directed us to a custom built home in the southwest part of town. While we were wandering around and commenting on a the beautiful post-war, French countryside look and pointing out the lovely cubby holes of libraries here and there, the real estate agent remarked: "What you really want is a library with a bedroom attached!" My answer, "Well, we do need *some* kind of kitchen." As it was, it was a house we both loved, precisely because of those little "library corners" as well as its beautiful style. So, books and reading material are very central to our lives and our relationship.

As time goes on, my husband still reads. A great deal. I have noticed in recent months that he reads more slowly and often has to sound out the words and, occasionally, gets them wrong. He still, however, reads. This I find amazing and I contribute his ability to maintain some independence to his constant search for new information. Sometimes his interpretation is a bit off the charts, but he still works hard at continuing to learn. The problem is he doesn't always remember what he has read. We do have a few subscriptions that come in the mail, however, when we are at the store he wants the current edition before his arrives. Sometimes we end up with two or more copies. Being a devout bibliophile myself, I have to admit that buying an extra copy or three of a particular magazine does not really bother me that much. He picks it out, it contains something he is interested in, and nothing in the world can convince me that there isn't room in the budget for this exercise. After all, even if my duplication is rarer I still spend a respectable chunk of our entertainment budget on books.

There are times when it is close to a payday and I have to ask him to wait, and I do mention from time to time that I believe we have a particular issue at home. He always waits if I mention a money constraint, but sometimes he is certain he does not have the issue so we buy it and move on. I do not purchase many books for him any more unless they are illustrated and address something he is trying to learn (or re-learn). Often, he feels as though he has to repay me for the things I am buying. It is these times when I point out that he is paying on his own credit lines, I'll just make a few adjustments. A few of the treasures I have found for myself end up on his shelves and I have to go looking for them and hide them while I am reading. I am learning that I must play nice and let him share: it's so much more peaceful that way.

The important point here is that whatever your loved one used to love, they most likely still do. If it is possible you should support some ongoing activity that keeps them occupied and interested. It's probably not a good idea to encourage bungee jumping, sky diving, skiing, car racing… but there should be something that you can bring into your lives that plays on that favorite interest or hobby. It is certainly suitable to work in the yard together (keep an eye on the equipment, it tends to move around a bit), go to museums or parks (as we have), or visit science centers or special events.

I have found that "getting out and about" helps me a great deal too. Usually, we pick something that looks mutually interesting and we take a camera. Yes, "we." I definitely try to get his buy-in when I decide on some outing. Not all plans work out, but some do and you have a moment to breath and see things in a different perspective. I know the afternoon I took him to the aeronautics museum in Calgary was really interesting for both of us. He assured me he knew many of the people talked about in the panels (probably not), he knew several of the planes on display (quite possibly), and he helped me pick out a few souvenirs. He still has his cup and will drink coffee from nothing else. Keep in mind, this was a respite for me as well. It was time away from the day to day struggles to enjoy something different, something of interest.

As odd as it may seem I have, on occasion, taken him with me when I have my hair done. If the beautician is comfortable with his presence, he actually enjoys watching how she works and creates something nice out of overgrown chaos. The point is that it is just as important for you to find outside things to do as it is for your loved one. It helps break up the stress of always giving care and adds a little sharing in the mix.

This was, actually, one of my awakenings after our return from the Island. I had been so focused on paying off our debt I left very little in our budget to enjoy ourselves. We are not young people with our whole lives ahead of us; at some point some of our hard earned funds needed to go toward something we enjoyed. Nothing extravagant, but certainly small, worthwhile projects would be acceptable. Invest in "time off" together; it really is important.

Movies and TV Shows

Another form of mutual entertainment is movies and TV shows. We have developed quite a collection of movies. Some he remembers. Some he does not. Sometimes he "remembers" things he could not possibly have seen. We also try to pick up on things that we will both enjoy when we are out shopping. That goal is not always met. I have noticed that when the subject is somewhat abstract or something that is sad or addresses death or war, he gets very agitated. For me this is difficult because there are movies without happy endings that I find of interest. As mentioned, I happen to enjoy watching M*A*S*H. However, whether it is because Korea was his version of a military service, or because he doesn't think war and mayhem belong in comedy, or even because the show was the favorite of a previous wife, he simply cannot tolerate it. The series in my opinion goes a long way to help us understand how we use humor to deal with the horror and terror of the world in which we live. This lesson is lost on a failing mind.

I do not recommend going out to movies. There is too much to consider with failing bladders, outspoken opinions, or the actions of other people. We did, on occasion, attend a Science Café in Calgary which presented a board of speakers on some selected topic. Finding programs that you enjoy watching at home does help keep people engaged and helps provide a routine of sorts for support. Usually we can find something along the lines of nature shows, or things about science and astronomy. History seems to be an acceptable subject if it is ancient history and doesn't involve war. He would not finish *Agora* although it addressed a point in history we had often discussed. Occasionally he will tire of a specific genre and we switch to something a bit different.

Recently he has developed difficulty getting all the way through a story that is more than, say, 90 minutes long. When it is something that I am actually interested in I do ask him if he minds if I finish watching. This works only if he doesn't happen to be going to bed. If that is the case then suddenly our living room is filled with people he doesn't know and he has to sneak to the bathroom or gets concerned about "that woman" sitting on the couch. Not really worth it. If I need to know how it ends I can find out some other way.

His tastes change and there are times when it is nearly impossible to keep up. My husband worked with robotics a substantial part of his career. Recently there were a few shows hosted by Stephen Hawkings about new discoveries. The first show was about the most fascinating advances in machine technology. Cars that drove themselves, wheelchairs that moved with the power of the mind, robots that learned. He thought it was all disgusting. I am not clear about what, exactly, was disgusting. We didn't finish the program. This, to me, is very sad because there was a day and time when he would absorb every grain of knowledge we could find from any source about developments in these areas of science. It is in these moments when I truly know that the man I met and married just isn't there anymore. It's always possible that it is the repetitive commercials and constant carnival hawking that bothers him. I think, however, when it is something that close to his career, he feels challenged, or bypassed, and becomes uneasy with the situation.

A close friend of ours had to stop television use all together because his wife could no longer tell the difference between real people and the people on the screen. Having a person with dementia watching television or other media is a bit like having children watching such things. Be sensitive to how much of it appears real to them and how much they understand to be a story. Sometimes that is very important and sometimes it is not. You are not educating a child, you are entertaining a failing mind. You do not, however, want something to add to agitation or cause difficulty in sleeping. If it is a scary movie and he or she believes that something bad will happen to the two of you; then you need to think about some other form of entertainment. If that interrupts your own viewing pleasure and you have an issue with that; then I recommend you get professional assistance and have a night out on your own. It really is not worth upsetting your loved one to watch some movie or program in part or in whole. If it is something important to you, take time out and watch it when he or she is not there or you are away from your home.

Through Thick & Thin & Emily Post

My husband has always been a thin person. He also has a metabolism that can consume several cups of sugar a day and, not only does he not gain weight, his blood sugar levels remain impervious to the onslaught. After his heart attack in 2005 we made some serious changes in our general diet. We were suddenly seekers of zero trans fats and, although I had always tended to healthier diet choices, we went into overdrive. The plan worked pretty well. Seven years and two stress tests later his heart health is still stable and there has been no further damage. These choices do sometimes limit a menu, especially during times of constrained finances. We developed a number of favorites that he would always eat, and a few things that he enjoyed, but not often. However, as his mind began to deteriorate, his appetite seemed to follow suit.

Somewhere in the year before his fall his appetite began to become quite a problem. He was losing weight and many of the things he had enjoyed before he now refused to eat. Of course, communicating at the store was more difficult when it came to picking out things he would eat. By the time we were well into the year after his fall I tried to make sure there were pictures to show him to see if he was really interested or if he was just going along with my choice to be nice. I really detest wasting food, so it was very important to me to figure out just what it was he would eat.

One of the tricks I learned is to watch when we went out to eat. His appetite was often quite good even if he could not finish the portion you usually get for an adult serving in a restaurant. My practice of using pictures did help to some extent. Ice cream was always a winner but I kept that back as a treat (he calls it a specialty). We also started to purchase a supplement drink (no advertising allowed in my little book) which helped keep his nourishment and his hydration up.

Liquids really are important in the health of an aging person. Dehydration can cause constipation, dizziness, headaches and other unwelcome effects. It is critical to keep fluids in aging people and you need to find enticing ways to do it. Elderly people tend to have less bladder control so they can and do avoid drinking a lot of fluid: not a good idea. Although I could often get him to drink water on a fairly regular basis, those supplement drinks in his favorite flavor really did it best. Of course, I had to be careful not to get the "improved" or "extra this or that" version, it had to be the one he had approved and accepted.

In recent months I have managed to change his diet enough that he has actually gained a few pounds back. It is important to me, but not always possible for others, to cook dinner and avoid prepared foods as much as I can. Steamers, rice cookers, slow cookers, five ingredient recipes, anything that makes it easy but also fresh. Read the contents. Some of those prepared meals do have low preservative, sodium and fat counts. Have a salad (not just iceberg and tomato), have breakfast for dinner, do things that make eating more interesting and you will get more input. And always remember that tastes do change and what works this week may not work in a month or two. I have also found that smaller but more often works well. Don't fix a large brunch and assume things are fine until dinner.

Eating alone does not work. My husband needs me at that table for at least part of the meal. This may make mid-day meals rather difficult since some people just can't be home during the lunch hour. Due to my ability to work at home (at least for now) I fix all three of our meals and I try to provide a mid afternoon snack. If you need to be away during some part of the day it would be greatly advisable to hire someone or find an accessible seniors' program to have a meal delivered. The things we tried included microwave preparation (both homemade and store bought), lunches in special places or bowls in the refrigerator (worked for a while) and leftovers redone for lunch (which also worked for a while). It is really important to watch and see if the food is being eaten, ignored or thrown away (so as not to disappoint you). A service that delivers a meal may have better success because it is ready to put on the table and eat. In our case, he would need to be well aware of the person and the reason for the delivery or the door would never get opened. Managing some sort of eating plan if you are not there is something you have to work with and tweak from time to time. Due to that "alone" part, it may be the best time of day to schedule a companion from time to time.

Finally, I have had to learn to deal with various ways of eating out. My husband has not liked eating around people for some time. It isn't really clear at this point why, although he seemed to think his chewing was too loud after he started using hearing aids. It may also be due to the natural withdrawal of a person on the path to dementia. Social situations are not the best place for insecure or confused minds.

What I do find now is that his choice of combinations may or may not be appetizing to other people present. I recommend that if you do eat in a group it is with friends who are as patient and understanding as you must be. It really is OK to put mint sauce on a salad, tea biscuits in your soup, gravy on strawberries or mix other ingredients in unexpected ways. You will not help your loved one eat right if you make the experience embarrassing or degrading. If they don't like the combination, well, maybe something can be salvaged that is edible. They may drool, a nose may run, things may not be so neat and tidy, but, oh well. The choice of utensils might seem odd, it becomes perfectly OK to eat sandwiches with a fork (or spoon) and knife. Keep in mind you are not applying for a job at Emily Post; you are caring for a loved one and his or her dietary needs. Keep a tissue box handy (for he or she to use, not you) and keep that person eating a reasonable diet at regular intervals in whatever comfort zone they need to accomplish that goal.

Emily Post aside, another aspect of dining is table setting. For years I cooked and my husband did the dishes. He also set the table and made sure appropriate condiments, sauces, dressings, whatever were placed on the table. At dinner it might be hit and miss because he didn't always know what I was going to prepare (neither, sometimes, did I). Thinking back it was probably during the last several months before his fall that I noticed a change. Salad dressing would appear at breakfast, syrup at dinner, spoons in the salad bowls, and other odd things. Obviously I didn't really pay too much attention to these odd habits, and I'm not sure it would have mattered if I had. Somehow I did know that it would not be a wise idea to correct, tease or get upset about the odd things happening. In fact, I think that the years we were "in between" we both needed the veil of denial, or our lives would have become a war zone. He would notice an error from time to time and apologize.

As time went on, these little chores deteriorated as well. He now helps with the dishes by bringing me things from the table. He has to find me before dinner and ask me what size plate (and how many) he should put on the table. We also end up with odd combinations of utensils and the condiments never leave the refrigerator. If he is given the juice container he will pour our drinks and I can hand him things from the refrigerator to put on the table. At some point during the day he usually pours us each a glass of wine, purportedly for dinner. It does appear to still be important to him that he contribute something. He is forever asking me to "show him how." And I do. As many times as he wants.

Grocery Shopping & Anything Goes

One of the things that my husband and I have always done when we were together is grocery shopping. Working through our budget, picking out things we would like to try, and formulating shopping lists so we don't get home and start the next one before the bags are empty, were all parts of our relationship. It was a process that we, quite frankly, enjoyed. We still do all of our shopping together, in part because I want his participation in order to get some buy-in on what he may or may not eat. There are a few things however, that have changed.

It was my practice to shop for two weeks at a time, basically securing the food budget out of my pay before the "if we have the money" things were dealt with. Since he always pushes the cart for me that has become a problem. The cart gets too heavy and he has difficulty maneuvering around corners. It seems like a simple thing but if you are trying to work through things together, provide stimulation whenever possible, and ensure that your loved one gets out and about now and then, these types of considerations enter into your planning. So, instead of one huge mountain of groceries every two weeks or so, we work at a trip once or twice a week. This also works nicely when you are trying to include lots of fresh vegetables and fruits in your diet.

Another duty my husband has always assumed was taking the groceries in to the house and putting them away. In part this was to allow me to soak a weary and sore back (caused by a childhood accident) and then prepare supper. Two problems have developed. I am no longer certain of his stability, and I tend to be a bit protective of his hernia repair, consequently I won't let him lift things that might be too heavy. Also, there is no guarantee where things will end up being put once they are in the house. Now we both unload the car.

During the year or so before the fall he would pop into the bathroom and ask me if something went "up or down." For some reason I was missing the fact that he no longer differentiated between a freezer and a refrigerator, according to him they could both have the same name. Not a major issue, I could rescue strawberries from the freezer and put frozen foods in the freezer while I was cooking dinner without really thinking about it. After all, I had found myself trying to put ice cream in the cupboard or tea in the freezer. But things definitely got more confused. About the time of "the fall" it appeared to me that it was safer for us both to put things away together. Then, one night, I forgot.

We were in the last week or so of the move from Calgary and things were in quite a bit of confusion. There were constant daily conversations about where things were (in a box), why (because we're moving), well, who took them? No one yet... I was trying to keep purchases to a bare minimum because when you cross international borders you cannot have open containers of any kind. So, because we needed laundry soap for a few more loads I purchased a different brand in a smaller container. It happened to be white. The next day while I was at work he called rather desperate. He had drunk something and it was just terrible. He could not tell me what it was nor how much he had drunk. Luckily it was close to time for me to go so I quickly drove home to try to figure out what it was he had done. He had used some of the "milk" in his coffee.

Not quite in panic mode I called the doctor and poison control and read the bottle. It is fairly evident that he had not ingested too much, after all it tasted pretty bad. The bottle itself said to give him lots of water; which I did. Apparently almost too much. A nurse later told me she still stuck to tried and true methods of inducing vomiting. Whatever the case we kept a close eye on things and he seemed to do just fine. After he realized what he had done, he felt rather foolish and apologized for causing such a turmoil. I, on the other hand, thought I had been rather stupid to not check just where it was that the groceries had gone the night before and considered the whole incident my fault. He had actually thought the white bottle was milk and had put it in the refrigerator; I never saw it until I got home the next day and he showed it to me.

You really have to be careful when you have someone in the house with a confused mind. It appears that they can usually determine what is safe to put in their mouth if such items are stored in the correct place. You do have to watch medications and keep a fairly close eye on alcohol consumption. For instance, there is little or no chance that my husband would have tried to drink laundry soap stored on top of the clothes washer. Another lesson in due diligence and awareness. Take a tour of your home and deliberately look for hazards or possible catastrophes. We no longer have throw rugs in some places, I make sure the tub has some sort of non-skid surface, and I help him into the shower. Use nightlights to avoid bumps in the night. Be aware of your surroundings and how they may impact a person who is not thinking clearly or may be less agile than he or she once was. The only long lasting effect of this adventure is that my dear husband no longer uses milk in his coffee.

Telephones That Translate & Other Tele-tales

Not too long ago my husband came to me somewhat distraught because the telephone we had in his office just didn't work. This seemed strange because he usually picked up that phone and listened to any conversation I might be having on an upstairs extension. He also thought I was calling him when it rang. So now it didn't work? What the problem appeared to be is that he could not reach the people he needed to. He took great pains to explain to me that he needed a phone that could speak different languages and would work at different times because, you know, it was a different time of day where "they" were. So, how does one solve this one?

After some thought it seemed to me that if I purchased a phone with speed dial buttons two things could be accomplished. My number would be available at the punch of a button and there would be no more concern about making sure that number was somewhere he would remember should he need me. Second, maybe there was a way to program each button to reach a different person in a different "country" and in a different "language." Don't laugh. What I was really working on is making sure there was a number or two he could dial to contact someone who knew him and would take the time to talk. What also happened is that his question sparked a whole different line of thought that included, hey, a speed dial might not be such a bad idea.

Initiating my new plan has had a few bumps. At first I told him I could only program the phone for him if I had phone numbers. Rather stupid of me, that doesn't satisfy him and it is obvious he wouldn't have any such numbers. One of those days when my mind was on something else like planting flowers or clearing the yard or something. Then, in an effort to get the phone to work the first day (while I was outside playing with those flowers), he unplugged it and didn't understand where the dial tone went. Explanations were again required, "Please don't unplug the phone."

Then, he wasn't happy about where the electrical outlet was because it interfered with pushing the cart the phone was on up against the wall (by a quarter inch or so). Couldn't I just move the outlet? Explanations of electricians, permits, holes in the wall and landlords that might not be happy...well, so what? Move the outlet. As it turns out our landlord might have been willing to do so. We'll have to wait and see if the subject comes up again.

What amazes me is that he figured out a configuration of his bookcases so that a small bookcase on casters fits between two taller bookcases and works as a credenza for the phone. This keeps cords from travelling from the wall to his desk and creating a trip hazard. So you see, there is still logic traveling randomly through that brain of his. I had started composing a list in my mind of persons that might be willing to go on speed dial, however he has apparently settled into the idea that the phone works. He can find the people he wants when he wants them; I don't want to rock the boat.

Arranging his office has been one of the things that keeps him busy from day to day. I just wish he didn't have book shelves nearly blocking the only exit door to the outside. Because he can see light and reach the handle to the sliding door he figures he has a path out, at least that's what he tells me. I suppose I should feel lucky, in our old house the basement did not have an exit to the outside at all and the windows were quite small or were made of very thick glass for privacy.

While on the subject of telephones it seems appropriate to discuss telephone conversations and lost etiquette. Until I had the direct line installed for the office I work for, I had to use our home phone for business calls. As noted, he would listen in from time to time. Often, I would hear him breathing on the other extension even though he said nothing. The conversation was beyond him and he denied listening. He told me that someone had called him and he wasn't sure why. The doctor's office has been instructed not to leave any messages at all because when they get him all I find out is that someone called and he doesn't know who or why.

We had a service in Canada that I truly appreciated and wish we had here. We were able to block our phone to any numbers that were not on a list that I programmed the service to recognize. That means no one could call and try to sell him a cruise or a better rate on his credit cards. This is a huge advantage to someone working with the elderly and really should be more widely used. I miss it terribly every time I answer our phone (which is on the do-not-disturb list) only to get a recorded message about some wonderful something or other that I can't live without. I have told him that if the caller does not say, "This is (my name)," hang up. Sometimes it works.

I also find that he has now developed a bit of possessiveness about his new phone. As I noted, somewhere along the line he managed to decide that it is, indeed, programmed for his purposes. When I call the house when I am away, he hurries to the upstairs so that he can answer the phone in my office; after all, I can't possibly talk to him on that "special" phone.

Every caregiver knows is it extremely difficult to talk on the phone with support services and doctors regarding the care of your loved one. Not only is there the possibility of the person picking up another extension and listening, they may be just around the corner and, with the aid of a sudden miracle, be able to hear clearly from more than two feet away. This is not a problem I have solved completely for myself. I do know that professionals and organizations that allow me to communicate by email and secure portals to the extent possible are a huge blessing. It is also an indicator to me that they understand the situation and may be able to come up with viable options for our situation. Another option is a cell phone that you can use when you go to get the mail or run some short errand that you manage without company.

Is it necessary to hide all this communication from your loved one? That depends on how aware he or she is of the condition and whether or not he or she is accepting or confrontational in discussions regarding a failing mind. My husband has given me enough evidence in the past that he would become quite confrontational and uncooperative should someone even suggest his mind is failing. Consequently, I avoid the subject as much as I can. This is one of the issues you must discuss with any professional support or facility. Everything you do can be undone in moments if a professional caregiver decides they *must* tell your loved one that they are losing their mind. Thanks, just what I needed, please go away while I try to pick up the pieces of my angry and devastated spouse.

It is so terribly important that you make sure that the professional help you seek is what you need and that the people you are sent are willing to follow your instructions or give you clear and acceptable answers as to why they must do something differently. As mentioned elsewhere; look for support resources that fit in *your* box, rather than surrendering everything to fit in theirs.

Ears & Other Removable Parts

My husband managed to put vanity aside and acquire a pair of hearing aids quite some time before we left for Canada. I think that I was able to convince him that he was missing a great deal. This was comparatively easy due to his love of classical music. There were parts of his favorite pieces that he just couldn't hear any more. I also noted that when he was tired the problem was much worse. In fact, some of our problems of one nature or another were because I would try to talk as I was walking away from him. A habit I still have and one that can be terribly frustrating to someone with a hearing problem. It's one of those "time" things. Does it take less time to stop, look the person in the face and communicate; or to have to turn around and repeat yourself in ever-increasing volumes?

For many years I blamed his failing memory on the probability that he simply had not heard and was too embarrassed to ask for things to be repeated. In part, this was probably true. As I have watched the deterioration of his hearing I have wondered if it isn't due, at least in part, to his inability to "hear" in his mind as well as through his ears. As it becomes more difficult to decipher the sounds you are hearing, it is also harder for the mind to interpret those sounds. It could have been a contributing factor to some of our misunderstandings. Did he really hear *and* understand what I was saying?

During a move from one home to another in Calgary that pair of hearing aids was misplaced. And although they were located many, many months later, we still had to deal with the issue of his hearing. So, after six months of realizing how much he missed them, we again went off for hearing tests. The new pair never seemed to work just right to suit him, but he did use them and often.

At some point in the months leading up to the fall he decided either that he didn't need them or they didn't work anymore. I think the biggest problem was that he didn't let the batteries activate before inserting them and they just didn't last or work quite right. I went over and over what had to be done, but somehow it was a procedure he forgot and never again remembered. So, I started to be the "fixer of the hearing aids" by replacing batteries, speaker domes and, eventually, making sure the battery door was in when he used them. This could pose a problem if something really was wrong with the unit so I also became a hearing aid tester. If I couldn't hear anything with them it was a sure thing he couldn't.

I am not sure when he started to confuse the function of the battery door. He started thinking that door should be open when the unit was in his ear. Occasionally he would put them away in the "ear house" and the batteries would be engaged making a faint squeaky-tweety sound that was just at the edge of *my* hearing. For me this was akin to chalk screeching across a chalkboard. So the process now included making sure the things got put to bed correctly. There are still times now when he insists there is nothing wrong with his hearing. "Yes, dear, I'll turn up the TV a bit louder." But if I ask in the right tone I can get him to wear them if we are, say, going to the doctor. I notice he uses them voluntarily much more often when they are working correctly.

As we age we acquire all sorts of extra parts and controlling the use and maintenance of these with a failing mind can get to be quite an adventure at times. For some years my husband has mentioned how "special" his shoes are. This in part because in Calgary, due to the mud and whatnot, one usually removes ones shoes when entering a home. He never would: his shoes were special. In this way they really were. Whether due to the composition of the soles or the tread he rarely tracked soil when he entered a house. These were also the shoes that we used as a base when he acquired orthotics.

For some years he has had trouble with his feet. Whether it is due to arthritis or other issues, there were times when his feet or toes hurt so badly he had difficulty walking. So, we went to a foot doctor and the orthotics were prescribed. Amazingly he did quite well once these were in those "magic" shoes. Now the exercise is, will he wear them? On occasion I find him in other types of shoes, shoes for slippers, slippers with broken down backs, but no nice, expensive, orthotics. And yet, when he does wear them, he doesn't have pain. It's another case of patient, continuous application of the, "would you try this," or "maybe this would help" kind of approach.

Since we haven't managed dentures just yet, the only other removable part my husband has to deal with is a hair piece. He has worn one since he was in his forties and, quite frankly, the style and type he wore did often make it difficult to know he wore one. It does make him look younger, although I would not be terribly upset if he suddenly decided not to bother any more. It used to be his practice to maintain and wear one each and every day even if he wasn't leaving the house. For him, it was part of getting dressed.

In some ways it still is; however his care of the pieces that he owns has deteriorated. He does not wear it each and every day, usually only when we are going somewhere or someone is coming. He also doesn't appear to understand all of the processes involved in cleaning and maintaining what he has. They are getting older now (as is he) and really need tender loving care. Enter care giving wife who spent time on the internet finding out the proper care and feeding of hair "systems." Another little chore on the list.

Unlearning to Drive

As I mentioned before, my husband suffered a compression fracture during a seizure that occurred while we were on our way to Canada. It took some six weeks for the fracture to heal to the point that he could start physiotherapy. To be quite frank, up until that time he was actually better at getting up and down than I was. This was of a great advantage to his healing. The sacrifice was that he had not driven for nearly three months and it took some gentle urging before we had him behind the wheel again. I took him out in the middle of a large shopping mall parking lot and let him get the feel of things again. Since we had only one car, I took the bus to work.

For most of our relationship I have done the driving. On some occasions for one reason or another, say, if I was sick, he would drive. He had become dependent, however, on my ability to find places without much ado or getting lost. He would often refer to me as his own private GPS. So, habits didn't change much through the years, and I still did most of the driving. During the years following his recovery he would not drive during the winter or at night. He would, however, meet me at the store after work or drive to the doctor's office near the bus stop where I would meet him. The walk from our house to the bus stop was several blocks and there came a time when he didn't want me walking so far in the dark and the cold so I started taking the car and parking in a park and ride lot closer to a bus stop. Then I made a major change.

For some reason I felt it was time I had the car closer to me during the day. It was also apparent that the time it took me to commute using public transportation was eating way too far into our day and was making him uneasy. So, in December of 2010 I asked my employer what was the best deal I could get on a parking spot. They let me try it for a few weeks without charge to see if it would really accomplish what I needed. The change was wonderful. Not only could I pick my path home, but I was able to come and go at slightly different times and avoid a lot of the commute traffic. This is why, when he fell that early January morning, I had a car within walking distance and could respond so quickly. Interestingly enough, I had just renewed his drivers' license from the state of Washington.

Giving advice on this particular "unlearning" experience is truly difficult. Some people know when they should no longer drive. My mother actually voluntarily gave up her car when it became apparent that she was too limited in her response time and driving opportunities. It is fortunate that my husband is so used to my driving that the transition has not been much of an issue. He does blurt out now and then that he could drive one place or another. He has offered to drive when I appear tired to him. But, occasionally, he will say something like, "Do you mind taking me? You know I'm not supposed to drive?" At least it has not come to a point of struggling over car keys and since he is not home alone with a car I have not taken his keys; he does, after all, still need to unlock doors. So, for the most part, we are admittedly dealing with this issue by not dealing with it. I sincerely feel for those who face struggles and battles over something so fraught with opportunity for disaster. In our society it is a badge of independence that is truly difficult to surrender.

There did come a time when I started dealing with the related issues. He was dropped from our auto insurance when we moved this time. It is also the first time I truly impacted his legal rights without his clear understanding of what was happening. As new residents in Washington, we had to update addresses and I had to change my driver's license from

Montana to Washington. Since we had to sit and wait for such a long time it seemed wise to take care of his license as well. The most important thing to me was that he had something in his wallet with his current address should an occasion arise that someone needed to know where he belonged. So, as we stood at the counter, and in his presence, I had his driver's license converted to a state ID card. I am sure that at his age they would have required either a written or driving test or both and it would have been apparent that he should not, under any circumstances, be driving. That, however, would be yet another blow to the fragile ego that lived with me and another opportunity for anger and rebellion. Thus, no license, no insurance, no driving. And I will find every excuse I can to make sure he does not get behind the wheel of a motor vehicle.

Recently, while talking to a professional agency, I mentioned that my current excuse was that we could not afford insurance for him just now. I have also made it clear we could not afford a second car. These excuses seem to work and avoid the impact of a clear statement of "you can't drive anymore." Seek an option that works, meaning, the one that keeps your loved one from behind the wheel of a car. Not only are you endangering your loved one, but there are other lives at stake for which you do not have the authority to make such decisions. If there is an accident and someone is seriously injured or dies do you really want to look them in the eye and say, "I didn't want to hurt his (or her) feelings?", or, "I couldn't face the arguments?"

Finances in Fantasy Land

How to handle finances when the mind begins to fail is the fodder of many, many late-night television shows and sometimes the pressure point for various legal and financial services to get your business early. It is, however, a crucial decision no matter how much you have, or owe, or how old you are. Sometime, somewhere, someone else will have to write the checks, find ways of meeting obligations or figure out the best way to use whatever resources were at your command.

In our situation, I have been managing my husband's finances in one way or other almost as long as I have known him. I helped him catch up on his tax returns, helped him manage his cash flow in an attempt to reduce his debt, helped him manage what small bits and pieces of treasures he had socked away toward the goal of survival. I had researched insurance plans, worked his credit card debt, churned his balances and set up monthly budgets to make sure his obligations were met. This, in many ways, has been helpful because there was no transition of authority, no moment when the reins of financial freedom transferred to my hands.

In recent years, however, it has become more difficult to manage some aspects of our "negative empire." Credit card companies do not like to talk to spouses about interest rates, they want to hear from the primary card holder. Since my husband cannot remember his social security number, phone number or address, that poses a problem. Some agents are very helpful when they understand the problem. Some, if they even get a hint that I am coaching, refuse to do anything. This, of course, is *not* helpful.

Should you face these types of issues and you are not the primary name on an account, you need to make legal arrangements that grant that authority. Yes, with enough intestinal fortitude you can probably bluff your way through, but if you are not completely supported by family or you do not have some legal document in place that indicates your loved one wanted you to handle these things, you could get yourself into a world of hurt. Plan ahead, way ahead, and know how you and your family want to see things handled.

The other part of handling finances is less legal and more a thing of perception. As noted from time to time in my little book, my husband lost the sense of money, where it came from and what it did. However, he seemed to be always conscious of whether or not he was contributing or whether or not someone on "my team" was helping. "I can't afford that" was a common issue. Or, "I want to pay for that." There were times when I would patiently go over things with him and explain that he did indeed contribute (he does receive social security and a small pension) and that he was not "living off of me (or my team)." It was also necessary, however, to continuously explain that we had to pay rent; that we couldn't afford a second car (whether we could or not), that we needed to wait in order to purchase certain things. He would ask permission to purchase a magazine or a book or some other thing; but then, without warning, some similar thought process would not compute.

He has lost the ability to understand the process of how I work, although he firmly believes that he is working. He has difficulty comprehending that by sitting in front of my computer 7-9 hours a day I earn money for our survival. When people call me he is certain it is about him and I must explain that it is someone I work with that is far away. Which, of course, also causes issues during those "right now this minute" events. As mentioned, during the months when I worked outside of our home he would often wonder how "those people" could be so mean as to keep me away for so long.

These are the things that take patience and are worth the time. You cannot deny access to things without some explanation of why. He or she may not remember the why, but if you fail to treat the person with respect, you will lose cooperation on just about any issue that has importance. You will become "that other" he or she that is not nice and is not supportive.

Another discussion we had over and over dealt with health care. It has been my considered opinion that both Canada and the United States needed to sit down in a big room and trade ideas (not insults) regarding the structure of a health care system. Both systems have their strong points, and both systems have huge pit falls. Much of the progress I made with my own health would have been impossible in the US because I simply would not have had access to the diagnostics I needed. My husband is, of course, on Medicare with a supplemental policy and his situation would have been far different. On the other side of the coin, in Canada I had to wait to get those diagnostics (as did he). In addition, our insurance came from the federal government and not the provincial. A number of providers had no clue as to how to access the program. Due to our status we could not pay and file for a refund. Either the provider accepted the coverage or we paid. But what coverage! I would not have had to worry about long-term care if we had been able to stay in Canada.

Eventually, we ended up as members of a private clinic. When my employer decided to change insurance providers the new underwriter would not cover my husband. This was because without provincial coverage we could not purchase the over-65 coverage that would support his prescriptions and assumed higher costs. My employer stepped in and, after I had conducted extensive research on alternatives, agreed to pay my husband's fee for the clinic. Due to this support, I had a whole team of people that looked for the specialists we needed. I didn't have to spend hours on the phone in a large room filled with cubicles trying to explain our status in Canada and how we were covered.

When this first happened my husband was still quite cognizant and understood, mostly, what a great gift this was. Looking back now I realize that he did not know how much of a struggle it was to find doctors willing to treat people who were not covered by standard provincial policies. He did not understand that getting to specialists demanded a referral and required waits, and sometimes money. He obviously did not realize how much pressure I had to apply to get him in for treatment when, for instance, he needed surgery to remove sinus polyps so that he could breath. The clinic took all that weight off of me and made it a private affair and not something every co-worker in a 20 foot radius would hear about.

If I look at the types of things we had arguments over in those last few years a lot of them had to do with medical matters. He would complain that he didn't like the doctor, or that someone at the clinic had said something terrible to him or about him or that he just didn't like that place. I would go over and over all of the reasons why the clinic was the best thing that could happen to us and how much they did and how hard they worked to take care of us. I would also point out that my employer was making this possible for us. He just couldn't put it together. It took me years to understand that it didn't really matter which government, which company, or if it was little green men from Venus that paid for our doctors. I needed to stick to the fact that the treatment he was receiving was covered without an undue financial burden on me (well, sort of).

Once we returned to the US there was a whole separate set of issues to deal with. Before actually leaving I had to make sure that his coverage was continuous. Our destination had a whole different set of rules for health coverage. So, I applied for him at a membership organization where he had been before. Things went fairly smoothly at first. They accepted my input for his medical history (which was an update on their files), prescriptions, current issues, family relationships and what not. But then I tried to change the phone number on his file. It looked like it was going to take an act of congress even though the number they had was an account that was in my name and no longer operative because it was a Canadian cell phone. How ridiculous to have my first real legal battle over the use of my own phone on a medical file! And, yet, there it was. Even with directives known to be on file, even with him standing beside me replying to questions in an obviously confused manner, it was a herculean task to accomplish that one goal.

Thus, another reason why you really, really, really need to have legal paperwork in place to fall back on when times get twisted. We managed, finally, to clear things up. In fact is was a very kind lady in customer service who simply asked him to sign a document that granted me access to his medical files for one year. He signed, happily, and we went our merry way.

This also brings up the question of long-term care insurance. I cannot, at this point, get insurance on my husband. Both because of his age and because he is already diagnosed with dementia. Of course, every company within a 100 mile radius is trying to get me to sign up at a time when my resources are devoted to caring for him. Without a crystal ball there is no way of knowing when it is time to invest in a policy that supports long-term care. What I can say is that all of my research indicates that if I was forced to place my husband in a home of any kind the annual cost would be near or even more than my salary range for the last five years. Not a happy thought. Medicaid is only available if you are willing to surrender assets. My mother's fairly brief stay (6-9 months) in a convalescent center has resulted in the assignment of the title to her mobile home at whatever time it becomes apparent that she can no longer live there. In the crazy quilt of regulations, insurance and care options inherent in the American system; it is critical that you at least try to be prepared.

Legally Speaking

That brings me to that real monster under the bed: legal status of persons with dementia and those who have to care for them. I was lucky, actually. In preparation for the surgery my husband had to remove those polyps I mentioned, we visited our attorney and asked that she draw up whatever documents were customary for persons living in Alberta. She set up the Personal Directives, Powers of Attorney and Wills for both of us with an alternate agent of his own choosing (who thankfully, accepted). As it happens, our doctor here in the States has accepted those directives as my husband's last known wishes and therefore good enough for him. The way in which our Directives are set up require the consultation of a medical doctor and a psychiatrist in order to have my husband (or myself) declared incompetent to manage his (or my) own affairs.

On the face of it, this seems simple. The problem arises when it becomes important to get that assessment. We almost managed at one point. As mentioned earlier in this tale, our doctor had set up a number of referrals to determine all of the implications of my husband's fall on that cold, January day. One of those referrals was to the Cognitive Assessment Centre at the University of Calgary. When our turn came up that fall I asked if a psychiatrist, rather than a neurologist, could make the assessment. This would fulfill the requirements of the directive. Yes, a psychiatrist could make the assessment and file the report. So, I set up the appointment and arranged to take the day off. I did not want to spend two or three hours having him bombarded with questions and then drive him home and dump him, most likely discouraged or even angry.

The eve of the appointment arrived, and, as we prepared for bed, he told me he didn't want to go. He didn't argue, get upset, talk about having no control or say he didn't like the doctor (whom he had never met). He just didn't want to go. When I later spoke with his son about the situation I told him I just couldn't bring myself to make him do what he obviously did not feel like doing. And, why? Just to make my life easier? And would it, in the end, make anything easier or would it have made him more aggressive, less cooperative? As it turned out we spent the day together, watching some special shows, shopping in an empty big box store (middle of the day, middle of the week), just being together.

Not all people have this option, if it was indeed an option. Many people in my situation have children, siblings, business partners, all sorts and kinds of persons in the world who do have, or feel they have, the right to decide what must happen in your life and that of your loved one. Sometimes this includes the impossible mountains to climb to handle medical care, credit lines, loans, ownership of real or personal property and a myriad of other issues. Each and every person must make their own decisions regarding how to handle what pieces they have to work with. The best advice I can provide is make sure that you and your spouse, parents, any family member make clear and make public what they want as life begins to fail.

A whole nation became involved in one case in recent years where the struggle was between a husband and the parents. We often hear of people unfairly committed with the ability to chose the course of their life stripped from them because of eccentricities, or different points of view. It is so very critical that your desires are recorded somewhere for future use.

It is also critical that you understand the legal implications of the choices you make. In reading about my obligations under the Canadian system I found some very good advice. Don't try to talk yourself into doing things that you honestly know the person under your care would not have done (say, spend all the money on a family vacation cottage and leave nothing for the care of your loved one). The book I read also warned against changing things such as beneficiaries on pensions or life insurance policies. Tinkering with the plans in place can severely weaken your case when you defend realistic actions under a trust agreement; which is, of course what a power of attorney is. I have, therefore, managed his funds as we have for years and, in fact, in a far more conservative manner. I do not use his credit to buy something fun for myself. I will use it to pay for subscriptions he has always had or to, say, fix a fire safe on the fly. Yes, I know he said he wasn't going to pay for it but I'm sorry, it *was* his fault I needed to go to such lengths. After all, *I* didn't lose the silly key!

Seek legal advice. Talk to each other while you still can. Understand the why behind your partner's or parent's decisions so that you can, in fact, act on their behalf as they would want. If you honestly believe that you cannot fulfill their wishes, you should discuss an alternative agent. Don't fool yourself into agreeing to do things you know in your heart you just can't do. When you make these choices and fulfill these wishes, do so in a manner that retains your loved one's dignity for as long as you can. It will go a long way to keeping him or her within the bounds of what you can manage.

Keep in mind, that sometimes you can't fulfill those wishes. A member of our family found it impossible to follow my grandmother's wish to be cremated. Her religious beliefs prevented it, and it was she and her husband who had been elected by my grandmother to handle her affairs. At the time my mother was pretty concerned that her mother's express wishes were not being followed. I told her that it was my feeling that funerals were for the living, not the dead and that if the issue was a matter of firm belief for this person, follow their desires. Grandmother had put her fate in their hands, let them make the decisions that no longer affected her directly.

The opposite was true in my father's case. I believe he was deathly afraid of being cremated (if you knew my father that statement would make sense). However, my mother's resources were very limited and a funeral with a casket and large scale burial would have put her further in debt. At the time I asked her, "Will you be comfortable with yourself knowing that you have gone against his wishes in this one aspect: or, can you be comfortable with a choice that will preserve something of the resources you have left? I will support either decision you make." She chose the more economic option.

Relationships With Real & "Real" People

One of the most difficult things for me to work with is my husband's deteriorating perception of people, real and imagined, who they are or what they do. It is the aspect in which I most often get caught solving the wrong problem. Sometimes I must reach quite far with creative answers to get him to move on and stop worrying about a perceived affront or an imagined expectation. Here are some of the issues we have faced.

There were times while we were still in Canada that I would set up a doctor's appointment and he would begin to fight me on going. Since we were signed up to a private clinic and it was not a simple matter to find another doctor I would come up with all kinds of reasons why he must go; sometimes I was reduced to tears. One afternoon, with a flash of insight, I decided to show him a picture of the doctor we were going to go see. Guess what, he liked that one; it's the "other" doctor that he didn't like. It was then that I began to understand that his confusion over who I was or was not could and did extend to some, not necessarily all, others.

From time to time he will tell me that someone that visits us on occasion, say, our landlord, doesn't like him. Maybe he will say the person said some unkind thing about himself or me. Sometimes he just doesn't like the person himself. And yet, the next time the person shows up he will be quite pleasant with them. At least once I heard him apologize to a person for an incorrect assessment (this would be the neighbor lady in Calgary during a good-bye tea).

Instead of arguing with him about whether or not that person may or may not say such a thing, or whether or not that person does or does not like him, I work to find some way to "take care of it." So, I might mention that if it (whatever that might be) happens again, let me know and I will take care of it. Sometimes he doesn't want me hurt or doesn't want me to suffer in any way, then I have to tell him, "Well, that's part of my job." I do not want to say I won't let the person come back because I honestly don't know if he has the person confused with someone else and if or when they do return I may lose credibility that I need to handle these types of situations.

It becomes a game of balancing what truthful thing I can say to handle the situation and still provide some reassurance that he shouldn't be bothered about this particular problem and that I am taking him seriously. In one case he informed me that the person that *said* he owned the house really owned only a small part of it. Really? He also has some idea that the person lives next to us over the fence or somewhere near. He actually lives a good half hour away.

It seems, but it's only a guess, that he suffers from some sense of insecurity so that if someone does not pay enough attention to him and his subject of the moment, they don't like him. Every person that comes to our house cannot devote special time to him, so I seek a balance, or mention something that I "heard." The point is not to get him to understand something other than what he thinks the truth is. That won't happen. You can, however, get the person to move on to another subject and hope to continue to defer the subject until it is no longer an issue. You can't however *not* deal with it at all and let it build. In that case he may burst out and say something that is totally out of context and, perhaps unkind. So, I reassure him that person X or Y is someone that is working for me and that, for now, this is the best deal I can work out, please be patient. If the problem continues we will look for something else. This reassures him that I am looking out for his side and, eventually, things smooth out.

There was a time when it wasn't quite so obvious that my husband was suffering from a deficiency and people would get caught up in a conversation with him suddenly realizing that things were a bit, well, not right. In some cases, people who come to do work in our home eventually get the idea they need him to "go find his wife." Since he loves to watch how people work and what they do he usually is right in the middle of things. So, when someone needs to know where something is or to convey some important information, well, I sometimes have to make sure that things are as they should be before a repair or service person leaves the house.

Many months before that fateful January morning my husband and I would get into arguments about people he met with during the day, people who were "in the neighborhood," people who called. As mentioned, our phone in Canada had a blocker on the system and unless I had programmed the phone number in or the caller knew an access code, they couldn't get through. When I would mention this I would get all kinds of creative explanations of how someone could bypass that system. When I doubted him, we argued. This behavior preceded his diagnosis by some time. Once we returned from Vancouver Island, I began to put some pieces together.

Recently, while watching a fascinating Science Channel program *The Wormhole* narrated by Morgan Freeman, we learned about some of the ways scientists are looking at the question of time. What it is, how we perceive it, whether or not it even really exists outside of our own perception. The program introduced an incredibly interesting individual named

David Eagleman, who has a Ph.D. in the neurosciences. His research indicates that many mental illnesses may be impacted by, if not caused by, the mind's perception of time. In the case of schizophrenia he believes that the problem is the patient's inability to correctly process time. Such a person cannot sort out cause and effect and has difficulty figuring out what things follow what actions.

I thought about that for a while and in some ways it did seem to fit. You see, as my husband's mind began to deteriorate, I became something of a forensic scientist. As he lost the ability to keep the walls he had built in his mind in place, I had a better sense of how those walls worked. He really was living in a house of mirrors and only the mirror he had lighted at any one moment had any existence in his mind: in that moment. This had to be the way he could, quite effectively, live different lives in such absolute honesty that his reactions to "discovering" something from another "life" was an obvious and very real surprise. Not quite a case of multiple personality, but similar results. So, as his mind began to unravel, so did much of what I knew about his past life. This, of course, is a subject best left for some later publication.

What this insight does provide at this point is the understanding that the people of his life tend to drift a bit and take on different roles in the history of his life. I know that his father lived until sometime in the 70s; however he has recently told me that he died in the attack on Pearl Harbor. My husband grew up in Hawaii, his family was there during the attack, but to the best of my previous knowledge he only lost a newborn baby sister. The event did seriously impact his family and their future relationships, but his father had survived.

Another "bleeding mirror" in the last few months involves his children. I knew of and had met his two sons. Recently, I kept hearing about four children, three boys and a girl. The only way that worked with what I knew of his history was if he counted the children of a woman he never admitted having married. He told a recent visitor he had 5 children. Then, no, the boys weren't really his. Well, her children weren't, but I'm certain that the two young men I met are. So, again, the details of his life are collapsing in on each other like some star going nova.

Even these people are "real." However, returning to the mysterious visitors of the months before that fall in January, I still find the most difficult part of this aspect of his disease is trying to come up with ways to deal with the people that aren't there at all. What does one *do* with all these extra people?

I should have known there was an increasing problem because there were many signs that pointed to this "bleeding mirror" affect. There were times before that January when he would complain that I was on the phone talking about him. It never made sense to me that he could "hear" me talking on the phone with my back to him or in another room but I had to speak directly in his ear for him to hear what I was saying in response to such a statement. I thought maybe I was talking in my sleep (*not* a good idea at this point). In tears I would sleep on the couch, pace the floor, sit up and drink tea, try to figure out what I was doing wrong. It became very clear as the deterioration became undeniably evident that the person speaking was not me, but someone in his mind. How do you handle such a thing as that?

After the fall this behavior got increasingly worse. There were times when he would get up in the middle of the night because someone was punching him. He would wander around in the house looking for people that were supposed to be there (or not). He started closing doors to various rooms, perhaps so he wouldn't worry about who might be there. He would ask me where these people went, when they were coming back, did I know who they were? Now he has special windows that he goes to in order to observe what is going on in our neighborhood.

You have to understand that simply telling your loved one that there is no one there will only anger them. Soon they will believe that you are "in on it" or that you don't want to tell them the truth. These were the reasons we would get in such arguments in those earlier months; I was trying to convince him of something he *knew* could not be true. Time for a new plan.

The way I handle this now is to approach it from the view that I did not see the person or persons. Maybe I was asleep, or I was busy, or in another room. They weren't expected, they didn't bother to tell me what they needed and, no, I have no idea when they are coming back, if ever. I certainly didn't invite them and don't particularly want them here. Notice that all of these statements do indeed have an element of truth, and, they do not challenge his perception of reality. You are not going to teach here. You will not find a way to logically explain it all away. You are maintaining a relationship in a manner that allows you to care for someone for as long as you can in the best way that you can without confrontation and emotional turmoil.

Sometimes this works. Sometimes he worries over it for hours and comes to me with any number of concerns about who these people were. Didn't I see them? No. Well, will they (he, she) be back? I sure hope not. Well, the car is there and it looks like ours. It is. And so it goes. It will not do for you to go look to see if someone is there. Your loved one must go. Turn on lights, keep the bed warm, walk with them if necessary but don't fight it. It does get wearing. Believe me. Especially if you are trying to do other things, like talk on the phone, work, read something important, actually watch the program you have selected to watch together, or sleep.

From everything I have read this problem of sorting real people from "people of the mind" is a symptom of dementia even if there were no prior issues of a similar nature. From what I am now able to ascertain, my husband has probably dealt with some version of the problem all his life; he just locked his characters, real and imagined in all those separate mirrors. The mirrors are breaking now, and all those characters have escaped into our home to haunt us in every corner. I do my best to keep them at peace.

Becoming Who I Am to Him

As mentioned here and there throughout this tale, I have become many, many people. Each and every day I practice shedding the skins of yesterday and try to put together who I am today. Some of these instances are rather humorous. Some are downright heartbreaking.

Shortly after our return from Vancouver Island, while I was still working most of the day in an office, conversations on the phone could take a bit of navigating. I, like most persons these days, worked in an office full of cubicles. When I would call to check on him he would want to know who was calling. So, I would try using my name, then, "your wife," then, as things got desperate, "the lady that fixed your breakfast." At some point I would give up and tell him I would explain when I got to his house. How this all sounded to my co-workers I have no idea; thankfully no one was making comments or giving me odd looks. It is still an issue that bedevils our conversations when I call. There are times when he recognizes someone that he is glad to hear from; and then I get home, and it wasn't me that called. I no longer try to keep track of this or try to convince him of anything. I simply check to make sure he is OK and express some desire to see him later.

There is also the issue of "home." Even now he will ask me if I am coming back, or if I will be "here" the next day. "Well, yes, I live here." That's nice. Or, he tells me it's OK to sleep with him (thank goodness for that, we only have one bed). He always seems to deal with me as who I am, but whoever that is doesn't seem to hold on to an existence for any predictable period of time. Even if I am in a different room than where he expects to find me he will wonder where "she" went and do I know when she is coming back. When I try to explain that it was me: no, it wasn't. Often I will get questions such as, "who are they going to send to replace you?" This morning, after sleeping with me all night, he expressed how glad he was to see me back, "Where did that other one go?" I had only stepped out of the room to put on a robe.

My personality has somehow split in his mind and I have become a whole team. Sometimes I am the leader and sometimes he wants to know if I need to report to someone. No, I don't. It would not be quite so difficult dealing with these multi-versions of myself if he didn't demand answers that I simply don't have. Why would he/she leave (I can be both). Why did he/she make me go there (because you wanted to). Who will take me to the doctor (that would be me). Who pays for us to stay here (yep, that's me, too). And on it goes, this moving sea of people that I am, but I'm not. It may be some part of those "broken mirrors" I mentioned, some unhinging of the pieces of me that reattached to some other memory or imaginary memory that he has. There are times when he takes me into his confidence and explains that "she" is jealous of me. Really, and why would that be?

Another event that caught me in an unguarded moment during that summer of change happened one afternoon when he came to me and said he had forgotten to ask me my name; and five minutes later, "I love you." So, maybe the Beatles had it right after all. He knew he cared. He just wasn't sure who it was he cared about.

One of the things I feel is really precious and somewhat odd is that he wants to marry me. He has asked several times and although I indicate that according to the laws of at least two countries we are married, well, no, we still need to get married. This started fairly soon after our arrival back from Vancouver Island. Our friends, the ones who were with us the first time, helped me arrange a re-commitment ceremony to see if that would put his mind at ease. It did, for a week or two. Now he suggests I find a minister so that we can get married. Perhaps somewhere deep inside his mind he still remembers telling me that he didn't want to be a burden for me to care for and he will not permit himself to believe that I still want him. Whatever the reason, it probably won't matter how many ceremonies I arrange, he will still want to marry me, or today's version of me. Which really isn't so bad. In fact it's rather cute.

There are times when he seems more precious to me than ever before. The instant mood changes seem to occur less often, I know it has been months since I spent the night weeping silently and wondering how to change his mood or his mind or at least my despair. Some years ago, a couple that I had been very close to experienced something of what I am going through. The wife in the marriage developed Alzheimer's. She actually was aware of the diagnosis and they worked together as a couple until her mental capacity would no longer permit it. He was by her side until the very end through many changes of home and geographical location. I remember giving him some advice one afternoon when she was not with us. I told him that the best way to survive what was coming was to realize that the woman he had loved all his life (they had been married for more than 50 years) was not there anymore. That in order to care for her and to survive his own emotional rollercoaster, he would have to grieve her loss and move forward with a different love. So, here we are, at the same doorstep. Did I take my own advice?

I think I have. In my own mind the man that I met and fell in love with is just not the person I now live with. He is gone and he will not come back. I ache for him, but I cannot care for *this* person if I focus on the person I have lost. So, this man, this precious fellow, is a man that I love with a different love. There are times when I experience a kind of flashback. Oddly, these are generated by watching his hands. I may be helping him shave or holding hands during a show, or holding his hand snuggled in bed and suddenly reality shifts and I see him as he was ten, fifteen years before. It is an act of will to pull myself back into the moment. I can no longer gaze into his eyes. Yes, I make eye contact. I don't avoid speaking directly to him. There was a time, however, when his eyes used to mesmerize me. Now they just remind me that a veil has fallen over his mind. There will be a time when I can treasure the memories that I have of our years together; but I cannot be a good spouse to the man I am now married too if I am forever longing for his predecessor.

Even with that separation in my own mind, our relationship is not built on what I think I can do for him or some gallant or misguided belief that I am somehow cosmically assigned to take care of him; it was built through years of helping each other cope, survive and succeed. He took care of me many, many times. He was at my side during years of migraines. He often drove me to hospitals and clinics for the narcotics I needed to control the pain. He would also get up often in the middle of the night to crush ice for me since it was the only thing that would stay down and keep me hydrated. He helped me manage my bi-polar condition by learning to see when the manic stage was starting so that it could be redirected and moderated and, thus, save me from the deeper dives into depression. He worked hard to help me deal with that depression. He also stood by my side whenever there was a doctor's appointment or screening. He encouraged me to reclaim my career and devoted many hours to reading manuscripts and papers he sincerely believed should be published.

Yes, there were things from my side as well. I listened, always listened. There were times when he was quite depressed, and I would not let him off the phone until I could hear his laugh. I believed him and I believed in him. That, of all things, was probably the greatest gift I could have given him. I could see, if only conceptually, what his mind conceived and of all the things left undone, his unfinished accomplishments in the fields he so loved are the greatest loss to me.

I was told while we were on that island that putting him on a plane that morning in May could have contributed to the acceleration of his illness. Evidently the change in pressure can affect certain medical issues within the brain. This is why people with recent brain surgery or tumors are told to avoid flying for some period of time. So what might have happened if I had listened to the vague uneasiness I felt that morning on the threshold of our dream vacation? If I had canceled everything and dashed him to the doctor could I have changed the course of his illness? Could I have purchased him a few more months of relative sanity? In the end I feel that even if we had preserved his then-current state of mind for two or four or six months it would have been at the cost of a week that we both had craved and needed. A week alone together among trees and mountains and on the shores of the Pacific Ocean; watching the surf crash against the rocks while talking of nothing in particular and everything in particular still within his grasp. At the point he had reached by that spring, nothing would have brought him back. But we still could share something precious to us both. Yes, I would do it again, even knowing what the impact might be for the future.

A number of people have told me that I now must make decisions that are best for me. What is often not considered is that many of the decisions that are best for him make things far, far easier for me. So, there is always a balance, one you must seek each day and that changes as surely as the speed and depth of the disease changes. This is why I call it a dance.

I hope our story helps others who have to face the loss of a loved one's mind and gives them tools to navigate through the days and months and years that may be left in each other's company. Know your own strengths. Don't compare yourself to others. There is a stanza in the Desiderata that goes something like this:

> "If you compare yourself with others,
> you may become vain or bitter,
> for always there will be greater
> and lesser persons than yourself."

I know that I have more energy than someone ten or fifteen years my senior; however I have to manage an outside job while I manage the job of caregiver. Perhaps the situation is more like a single mother, who, ten or fifteen years my junior, would have more energy, but perhaps fewer resources or less earning power. There is no way to gauge one person's ability to carry a burden over another's. So don't try. Take each day as it comes and make the decisions you must for the safety and well being of yourself and the one you love.

I wish you well on your journey, whatever path you follow and

> "... be at peace with God,
> whatever you conceive Him to be.
> And whatever your labors and aspirations,
> in the noisy confusion of life,
> keep peace in your soul."

Made in the USA
Lexington, KY
08 June 2013